If it isn't **FUN**, it **ISN'T** fun.

Teach Your Child to Talk Faster Than Speech Therapy

From the mind of,

Marci Melzer, M.Ed./SLP
Intuitive, Speech-Language Pathologist
Language Facilitation Consultant

Copyright © 2019 by MM SLP Services, Inc.
All rights reserved. This book or any portion thereof
may not be reproduced or used in any manner whatsoever
without the express written permission of the publisher
except for the use of brief quotations in a book review.
Printed in the United States of America

ISBN 9781694063229

Independently Published

www.WavesofCommunication.com

This book is written as part of my mission to help as many parents as possible, teach their late-talking children how to use the words they need to share their wisdom with the world.

Table of Contents

Forward 7
Getting Ready for Your Language Facilitation Journey 22
What is Really Going On 40
Helping Your Child Overcome Resistance to Talking 53
Waves of Communication Results the First 20 Months 65
What's Blocking Your Child's Speech? 67
Reach and Teach Your Child the Words They Need 93
If it isn't FUN, it ISN'T fun. 112
Online Resources to Support Your Language Facilitation Journey
.... 117
About the Author 119
Are You Ready to See FAST Progress? 121

Forward

Why did I write this book?

I have been guided by my own intuition, to share with you how powerful you are. I have proven that parents can teach late-talking children to use words naturally, and faster than any professional, even the best speech therapists. I have learned that it is important, and indeed necessary, for parents and therapists to use their natural intuitive abilities to help the late talkers in their lives learn to use language naturally.

My name is Marci Melzer and I am an intuitive speech-language pathologist and language facilitation consultant and coach.

The systems currently in place in our world to help speech-delayed children learn to talk are broken and they are creating fear and worry in parents that is not necessary. I have found a better way for parents to help their children learn to talk that is proving to be way more effective and a lot more FUN.

My journey to gain the knowledge I am sharing has been long and winding. I worked all over the USA as a contractor speech-language pathologist/therapist for 29 years. First, I worked for agencies and eventually I worked as an independent speech therapy service provider. Every year, I was assigned to a new placement and many years I worked in more than one facility.

Contractor speech pathologists are used when a school, health care center, hospital, or clinic, can't find their own therapist or don't have enough work to hire one full time. We usually get the worst schools in the district, the hospitals with the poorest facilities, and the families who live in the roughest neighborhoods. Contractors get the assignments that other speech therapists have turned down.

Why did I do that for so many years... and why did I leave?

I have eventually discovered the real reason I moved around so much is that I was learning. It felt like searching for the right place/job for me to fit in and be happy long term, but I never found true happiness real effect on the world when I was working in any of these "systems" that I was placed in. Every placement had so many hoops to jump through just to be able to work with families! There were always the same politics within the facility surrounding making money or cutting costs.

There were always extra responsibilities of extensive data collection and reporting. There was also a lot of stress placed on therapists for meeting productivity standards and seeing "enough" clients to meet the government standards AND making enough money for the facility stay within budget. I had no control over the clients who saw me, and the clients had no say in their process either. All these issues and responsibilities took away from the time and energy I needed to provide effective therapy and the whole process left me exhausted and my clients frustrated!

I always left each assignment with a feeling of relief and hope that the next placement would be better. Unfortunately, it never happened for me and it is the current reality for most speech therapists working today.

The most recent and rapidly growing money-making trend the system has created, is to get as many clients as possible to be "diagnosed" with autism. This is the healthcare business world's latest boon and it is being abused by all kinds of providers, all over the world. It's no secret that the global insurance and government systems which fund healthcare globally (including speech therapy) are currently paying for "services" only when children have received an "autism" or "autism spectrum disorder" (ASD) diagnosis.

This trend is the reason I left speech therapy completely. I tried to avoid being part of it, keeping silent as the obvious bias toward getting more kids diagnosed with autism was "encouraged" by the government programs, schools, and even the American Speech and Hearing Association which is the governing agency for speech therapists.

The final straw happened when I was presented with a contract that I could not ethically sign.

This contract was presented to me by the government-funded early intervention program in the state of Florida, USA and it had a stipulation that ALL early interventionists are required to refer every child older than 9 months of age who displays even "subtle characteristics" of autism for a formal autism screening.

They had provided in the previous year's contract 30 hours of mandatory "autism identification training" to clearly educate all providers on the subtle signs of autism and how even babies can show these signs. This next contract would require all those who completed the training to start referring more children.

Of course, being a speech therapist, every child who would be assigned to work with me, would display the primary "autism characteristic" indicated on most checklists and highlighted in the training videos - speech delay. This contract would require me to refer every client on my caseload for autism screening/evaluation just for the purpose of getting more autism diagnosis on the books.

I know, from working with thousands of speech-delayed children, that they almost always display characteristics that fall on those autism checklists. I also know that when a complete history is evaluated, there is clear evidence that the speech delay is caused by one or more other conditions. A few very common causes of speech delay that look a lot like autism are hearing loss, even temporary due to ear fluid, technology addiction, and vision problems.

This broken system is spreading all over the world. This is evidenced as parents report to me almost daily that their doctor has given to their child (or offered) an autism diagnosis even when TRUE autism is not clear. The children may have no other clear and consistent symptoms except late talking, and doctors are still giving autism diagnosis just so parents can get "services" from government agencies. Parents are also often told that the diagnosis can be removed later if the child develops the "lacking" skills.

Parents and kids are the victims in this system. What's happening is that providers encourage parents to get doctors to misdiagnose their children so they can sell more therapy.

It is very common practice and freely communicated by parents all over social media that they go to the doctor requesting an autism diagnosis just so they can "get services." I have read many blog posts about parents giving their kids medications, so they appear more "disabled" than they are, and they are. This is clearly blatant and technically fraudulent misdiagnosis for the purpose of working the system because of money.

Parents always have access to services from speech therapists without a medical diagnosis, they simply need to pay for them out of pocket. But therapy is expensive, and the economic status of MOST families worldwide simply does not allow for this expense. Parents are left without any other option than to lie, cheat, and literally steal funding to pay for these services and find help for their nonverbal kids.

If you are reading this book, you likely have a late talker in your life. It is also very likely that you have also experienced at least one professional "suggest" or "suspect" that your child has autism - with or without a formal evaluation. If you have been referred for early intervention in the United States or seen a speech therapist who works for some kind of public facility or school, it is very likely that your clinician will bring up autism referral and your child will end up with an autism diagnosis by the time they go to elementary school.

This is true even if you, as parents, have never considered that your smart, interactive, curious and late-talking child could possibly have autism. It's a very big problem too, because children who are misdiagnosed are potentially at risk of real, long-lasting emotional and physical harm.

Misdiagnosis completely stops investigation into the REAL cause of the child's issues.

Speech delay can be caused by hundreds of factors. If the TRUE underlying cause is not properly identified, then the actual physical problem could worsen without the most appropriate treatment. I have observed many cases where, after mild autism was diagnosed, children were found to have had hearing loss significant enough to delay speech and/or vision difficulties that prohibited them seeing peoples faces. In each of these cases, the parents were hurried into getting an autism diagnosis and starting ABA therapy, before their child was 3 years old.

Each case resulted in highly frustrated children who were unable to see or hear well enough to comply with the requests. Their anxiety caused them to have increased behaviors and their mild autism diagnosis was elevated to moderate or severe. In each case, when parents removed the child from highly structured therapy and the vision and/or hearing issues were corrected, the behaviors went away, and the children learned to use spoken language very quickly.

I believe intensive intervention like ABA or PROMPT therapy cannot ethically be prescribed by a practitioner unless they are 100% positive of the autism or apraxia diagnosis. These therapies can be highly invasive to a late-talking child. They require frequent sessions of repetitive tasks that cause many late-talking children to develop anxiety. There is no 100% accurate diagnostic measure, like a blood test, that can prove a child has either autism or apraxia. In fact, the diagnostic measures used for applying these labels each rely on a child to actively participate in the evaluation process.

So, a child who is unwilling to participate is, by design of the test, judged by the evaluator. The evaluator's responsibility is to determine if the child is TRULY unable to complete the task. The same is true when speech therapists diagnose speech apraxia in children under 3-years-old. The American Speech and Hearing Association advocates comprehensive and dynamic evaluation including oral motor assessments that little kids can't follow. Speech therapists who specialize in treating either autism or apraxia are biased by their experience to look for these conditions. Therapists with professional bias are quick to diagnose a child before they have completed comprehensive language testing and long-term intervention as well as extensive parent interview and review of the child's entire developmental history.

Perhaps you have had a therapist or doctor tell you that they "suspect" your child has apraxia or that your child may be "on the spectrum" of autism, however, the evaluator can't confirm for absolute sure. Many parents report that they have been instructed to initiate ABA therapy by their medical doctor even when the doctor tells the parents that they don't think the child even has autism. Any intervention taken to address a "suspected" diagnosis is a simply a guess to resolve the problem. Without proper diagnosis, even the therapist can't know WHY they are doing the intervention! They are simply using the therapy to train skills that will compensate for the symptoms they see.

Misdiagnosis is a bad idea because the "services" or "prescribed treatment" that go with autism diagnosis are designed for those who truly do have that diagnosis. Would you want your doctor to misdiagnose your child with a medical condition if the treatment was invasive drugs that could potentially harm them?

Many "seemingly" noninvasive interventions, including behavioral therapies and nutritional protocols that show "evidence" to "help autism symptoms" also have side effects to the child's mental, emotional, and even physical wellbeing that may create significant anxiety and stress in children both with and without autism. I have observed and reported abusive behavior toward children in public and private therapy environments and instances are reported daily in the media. Parents I work with have reported their children's increase in autism characteristics after beginning behavior-based therapies.

Think about it, with so many children being labeled as autistic and the number consistently rising how can one "protocol" or "method" help EVERY child with that diagnosis? How could every different child with very different unique special needs find real success in the same kind of intervention? It's just not possible, still a system is created around it and parents are being duped.

Unfortunately, even after hundreds or thousands of dollars on evaluations and intervention, so often parents are left without any real information or plan on how to help their kids. No parent should be expected to blindly accept, pay for, and implement a prescribed treatment based on a guessed or "suspected" diagnosis. Still, this is what the system expects of parents who have late-talking children.

What's worse is that parents continue to struggle to get through the days with their kids for years without any real progress. Unfortunately, as bad as the misdiagnosis problem is, the system has created a bigger problem and it is all to perpetuate the money flow into the system. The therapy is designed to keep kids stuck in these services instead of helping them succeed functionally.

Therapy companies, insurance companies, and the government tax programs only make money if they show that more kids need more therapy. So, the system needs to prove that the therapies paid for by these funds show "progress" while keeping kids coming back week after week for the rest of their lives!

The reported evidence that proves these therapies are "working" comes from data collected while the child is doing the therapy activities. In speech therapy, the child is trained to do a skill that can be measured (usually to say a word) and then the child is asked to do that exact skill repeatedly (say the word multiple times, or say all the words in the therapist's list) then the responses are recorded and reported. To get the child to try to do the skill, the therapist will use a positive reinforcement like a toy, bubbles, or food. The child identifies the skill (saying the word) with the reinforcement (bubbles) and they learn to do the skill when they are asked, understanding that the reward is coming. It is easy to count how many times a child says a word when asked, so it is easy to collect data.

Kids usually learn to say words quickly when the words are easy enough and the reward is great enough. So, it is relatively easy for therapists to get kids to say more words with this method. Because this repetition method usually words great for therapists, parents are encouraged to try it at home as well. So, they start to hold back the things their child wants and ask them to say words like the therapist does. Soon, everyone in the child's world is asking them to say words and repeat words.

If this is done frequently enough, the child will learn to say words to get the things they want. The number of words that the child can "say" goes up and that looks like progress. In fact, this question "How many words does your child say regularly?" is the standard measure by which many doctors screen children for speech delay, and document progress in their developmental screening measures. You have likely been asked this question by every person who has evaluated your child.

<u>*Here is what none of those professionals are telling you.*</u>

Saying words in response to a prompt, just to get a reward, is a memorized behavior. It conveys the same message as a gesture, like pointing or handing someone a picture. When kids need prompts to talk, this is not independent spoken language, and all of those words they say are not speech. Kids are saying words to make you give them what they want, in the moment, and they are not learning how to use these words functionally.

This is why so many families report that they have been in speech therapy for months, or even years, and their children are "making progress" and saying lots of words, but there is very little actual verbal communication going on. In fact, many children develop increased social anxiety because their speech is not functional for social communication. The process teaches kids to be MORE dependent on others, because they learn to talk only when prompted.

That is because while all adults are using this teaching words and prompting method with the child, nobody is facilitating natural, conversational language! Human brains are developed to learn spoken language. That's what makes us human. We are evolved as a species to learn spoken language naturally, from listening to our parents as they care for and raise us.

The frustration caused by relentless prompting and nagging from parents to say words causes kids to STOP listening to them, which blocks progress! Parents in my program have proven that when parents do stop prompting their children to say words and facilitate natural language, their kids develop the ability to USE the words they have memorized to say what is on THEIR mind.

If prompting persists without natural language facilitation, late-talking children may learn to say words to communicate needs and for their own entertainment, however, their primary communication of emotions and independent ideas continues to be expressed through nonverbal behaviors.

These behaviors are how parents primarily understand their children's needs and it is from these behaviors that parents know what words to prompt them to say. People who do not know the child intimately will typically not be able to understand all the subtle communication behaviors that late-talking kids use. In fact, behaviors used for communication as well as frustration behaviors may increase as children get older because their memorized vocabulary falls far short of their communication needs.

Often, parents of older children are guided to use a computer device. Their kids have increasing behaviors and they are still not effectively communicating after tons of therapy. Often, at this stage, speech therapists are spending all the therapy time programming and training children to use computer devices and facilitating natural verbal speech is no longer a goal of the therapy. The behaviors continue, requiring more and more therapy to manage and control them, the computer device is a whole new learning process, requiring a whole new course of speech therapy, and the child never develops natural spoken language because nobody is facilitating it.

The most important take-away from this information

If your child can hear spoken language, they can learn to use some level of independent spoken language naturally from their parents. This is true no matter what the root cause of the speech delay is, no matter what the diagnosis. I have proven it with more than 60 families living in 12 countries, many who are bilingual.

How I Developed My Language Facilitation Training Process

Over the years I have worked with people of all ages to facilitate speech, language and swallowing in hospitals, nursing homes, clinics, residential facilities and just about every kind of public and private school. My favorite work by far was when I worked with children in their homes because I could work in the family's environment where they are most comfortable. Most recently, I was contracted to provide speech therapy in the Florida State Early Intervention Program. I was directed by the program to use a coaching model and train parents to help their children learn to talk.

Some parents were not interested in receiving coaching on how to facilitate language with their kids themselves. They just wanted me to show up and "fix" their child's speech and language. So, for these kids that is what I did. As hard as I tried to share information, these parents didn't really want to hear about the session, they just relied on me to do all the work and didn't care how I did it. Those kids whose parents were not involved in the language facilitation process, always made the slowest progress.

Other parents were excited about working with me. When I met them, they had been searching online for strategies and were they were already trying really hard to work with their kids. However, they were finding that the typical speech therapy tricks and tips for parents they read online were not working. Their kids would go away every time they try to do any teaching. The same problem was happening with my speech therapy. In most cases, the kids would love to play with me. I could easily get them to engage with me and my bag of toys. I could easily facilitate sounds and words sometimes within the first few sessions. But, when parents tried to do what I did themselves in between sessions, their kids enjoyed the activity, but as soon as it looked like teaching… they quit.

So, I knew that the children have potential for learning to talk, however something was blocking the "teaching" process for their parents. I also knew that if I could help these highly motivated moms to use their strategies more effectively, their kids would be getting effective language facilitation all day and could make much faster progress.

I started to spend time during my sessions observing parents doing everyday tasks and playing with their kids so I could analyze the language facilitation situations from the late-talking child's perspective. I looked for what was different between how the child responded to the parent and how the child responded to me when we were playing with the same toy. I looked for the triggers that either made the child happy or caused the child to shift their energy and attention away from the parent.

Every family was different, however, each one demonstrated clear patterns of how they "work through" communication in their home. In fact, each child had trained their parents to understand their own unique "language" comprised of a combination of nonverbal methods such as gestures, demonstrations, pantomime, facial expressions, sounds or screaming, behaviors, and telepathic intuitive communication, sprinkled with memorized words and echolalia. Late-talkers try hard to communicate ALL of their needs, feelings, and cool ideas via this nonverbal language. If parents don't understand them, they try harder to communicate their ideas nonverbally. I observed most late-talkers and their parents to be stuck in this pattern. No matter how many words the child learned, their go-to communication on a day-to-day basis was all behaviors.

The biggest trait that I observed in every late talker is that they LOVE when their parents say the words for the things they are demonstrating. This is because sharing ideas between people is why kids, and everybody human, wants to learn to use spoken language. People don't need any reward to want to tell people our feelings, the reward comes when someone understands us, helps us, shares our feelings, and empathizes with us. Therefore, we have evolved the ability to learn and use spoken language.

Even simple animals can communicate basic needs nonverbally. Early linguists such as Noam Chomsky discussed that humans are the only animals that have the ability to use spoken language, and we evolved to use it for social communication. I believe that subconsciously, children know they need to listen to their mothers talking to learn how to use speech functionally.

Children did respond to directions and imitate FUN nonverbal actions that they enjoy without hesitation, especially when they were demonstrated by their parents. The children were able to learn nonverbal tasks that they enjoyed very quickly with only a few tries and the child even asked to try the skill again if they were having fun. Alternatively, there were a few instances that always sent the child away.

First, if the child perceived that the activity was too challenging and the parent was not helping, the child refused. Second, If the child was trying to direct the activity and the parent took control, the child shut down. Third, If the child was not independently focused on the activity, they did not participate, even if the parent made them sit in one place. The child just sat and endured the time obediently or struggled until released without any actual learning taking place. Another interesting observation was that most of the time, when parents prompted kids to say words, the kids were not even listening. Parents had to repeat the request at least 2-3 times for the child to respond, unless it was a highly preferred object.

After my analysis, I decided to shift the way I was working with families. I shifted to coaching parents in the exact methods to help them eliminate prompting and model the words their kids want to hear. I also gave them specific strategies to facilitate speech and language with FUN during their personal everyday activities like getting dressed, eating and riding in the car.

I also helped them replace their child's communication behaviors with words. This way the parents learned strategies to solve the speech and behavior problems they are most concerned about in their home. The parents were highly motivated to solve these problems, the strategies were FUN and it worked!

Then the system broke for me and left the system of speech therapy forever. I started studying energy healing and developed my own intuitive abilities. I also realized that years of working in a broken system had taken a toll on my own body. After two years of physical, mental and emotional healing, my mission became clear.

I was guided to start my own platform called Waves of Communication to reach and teach families of late-talking children all over the world and empower parents everywhere to do the language facilitation themselves.

I have seen thousands of late-talking children who all desperately want to use verbal speech. I have seen many kids stuck for years in nonverbal patterns because their parents don't, won't, or feel like they can't teach them. I have also seen enlightened parents find their nonverbal 5-year-old's children's speech in the first week. I have been able to work with families all over the world by empowering them as parents use the intuitive knowledge that they automatically have to understand what their kids resistance to using words is all about and then how to overcome those issues and enjoy playing with and functionally using speech and language every day.

Because the bottom line is that, when you can help your kids to overcome their hesitation to try words and make speech and language learning fun and happy, your child will start to talk. Think about all the things you have already taught them! Now you can facilitate language when you harness the natural intuitive knowledge and connection that you have with your child. It is incredibly powerful.

There is one more piece of the puzzle that every parent should know. Late-talkers, just like all kids, want to make their parents happy. They want to see you happy because when the Mom is happy the household is happy. Parents are responsible for keeping the energy of the household balanced so everybody can communicate effectively. Late-talking kids can perceive when their parents are worried, anxious, or fearful of the future.

So, if you are feeling worried a lot, your mindset needs to change for language facilitation to work. You need to focus on the potential of your child's talking and take the right action every day. All strategies must be easy, happy, safe, and fun for children and for parents. This keeps the energy positive and happy for all.

When these kids start to use language, their whole household changes. When these kids start to use words successfully, they give up all the behaviors that were replacing the verbal communication. They give up the tantrums, whining, hitting and screaming because they understand that words are easier and make the whole household happier and calmer. It is amazing to see parents all over the world literally change the energy in their household while they teach their children to communicate. This happiness radiates out from every family that overcomes their worry by solving their problems. This conversion of low energy (worry) to high energy (happiness) helps heal what's uneasy in our world.

It's my mission to help parents teach their late-talking children how to use the words they need to share their wisdom and help heal the world. I have figured out how to teach parents to use their own intuitive connection with their kids to help them to solve communication problems and find their child's speech naturally, in their own ways, in their own homes and see the improvement in their child's communication naturally occur throughout their lifetime together. Keep reading to learn how you can make it happen in your life.

Getting Ready for Your Language Facilitation Journey

Now is your time to take your child's communication in a whole new direction toward spontaneous verbal speech. You're headed down the path of your language facilitation journey and in this first phase you're going to need to get ready.

In this chapter I'm going to discuss with you: Who language facilitation is designed for; the criteria necessary for a child to start talking quickly with language facilitation; and the secrets for success with language facilitation.

Who is Language Facilitation Designed For?

Language Facilitation, and my Waves of Communication resources are designed for parents who truly believe that your children have the words inside, and that your children want to talk. It's for parents who know their child better than anyone. Parents who are ready to consciously examine their current intervention methods and stop any methods that are blocking your child's language development. Language facilitation is for parents who are willing to take responsibility for their role in the current situation. Not just how you got here, but how you're going to get out. This program is for parents who are prepared to invest time and energy into targeted language facilitation every day. You really need to take action to see results. Language facilitation is for parents who want to have fun during the whole process.

With an explanation like that, it may seem like there will be a lot of extra things to do. In fact, the opposite is true. With language facilitation, you will be eliminating most of the "therapy homework" jobs and replacing difficult and confusing strategies with natural, easy, and fun opportunities to teach your child naturally. The biggest effort in this whole process is deciding to make a change. After that, the whole process becomes easier every day and a LOT more fun. The language facilitation journey is for parents who want to have FUN and be happy with their kids while they teach them to talk.

The language facilitation journey is for parents who are ready to make the changes needed to see a different outcome. This path is not for parents who make excuses for their lack of willingness to change themselves. If you want to experience a different outcome, then you must change your effort. This is true for everything we experience in life. The truth is, there are habits going on in your household that are blocking your child's speech and you are the only one that can facilitate the habits of your household. Without change, the blockages will continue and either delay or prevent completely your child's natural speech development.

The language facilitation journey is for parents who want to help their child WANT to learn language from them instead of forcing them, begging them, or bribing them to do so. You know your child must change too. They need to switch from being totally comfortable and happy in using their made-up nonverbal communication systems to wanting to and consciously trying to learn to talk. You must help your child become motivated to stop relying on you to communicate their messages for them and want to learn to talk themselves. You can't force the changes or make any excuses about inability to change. You must understand what habits need to be changed and take new, correct action that you are SURE will take you toward the outcome you are searching for.

This process requires parents to identify and celebrate every super-cool thing your child does to empower them to feel like MORE than the other kids on the planet. You know your child is a superhero and they have superpowers. Their superpowers are the things they love doing and that they have learned to do well. Maybe it is running, doing puzzles, taking things apart, memorizing, spelling and/or reading, eating massive amounts, or doing math and navigating online video platforms. Nonverbal kids often have many extraordinary talents. Language facilitator parents learn to use a child's superpowers to offer interesting and fun opportunities to teach language.

Language Facilitation requires parents give up negative mindset habits. This journey will be challenging for parents who complain about their child's physical diagnosis, symptoms, and/or behavior; blame their life circumstances, or react in a negative or harsh manner to other people's opinions. You need to start considering all of the input you receive as objective information and make decisions based on what YOU know to be true. You oversee your child's world and you know them best.

In our world, it is commonplace for people to freely share their opinions and judge things and you can't stop this from happening. What is important to remember is that you always do have control and you are always in charge of how YOU feel and react. Your mindset goal should be to objectively evaluate the things other people tell you and decide for yourself what is right and what you and your family. Consciously forgive the people who don't understand your child and release that bad energy which is blocking your progress.

There are many common mindset traps that parents of late-talking children fall into as they navigate through the challenges in your life. If you're constantly worrying how your child compares to any other kids, looking up checklists about what kids should be doing at what age, and asking others their opinions about your child, then the language facilitation journey will be long and frustrating.

These habits of worry about the future and victim feelings of lack and loss are negative reflections on your child, and your child perceives them. Negative-thinking mindset habits also take your conscious effort away from helping your child move forward. They literally waste your time and energy and keep you stuck and unable to take the action you need to make the changes required.

You will need to be responsible for keeping your focus on ALL the positive things your child does to encourage them to make the hard changes. Every child is amazing at something. Language facilitation is for parents who refuse to believe it requires a professional therapist or teacher or doctor to help their child talk. Many kids are late-talking due to physical, biological, and systemic issues with their body. Parents definitely need to work with the appropriate holistic physical intervention on keeping their child healthy but being physically healthy alone is not enough to help your child start talking. Parents must incorporate focused language facilitation strategies on top of keeping your child healthy to get them to teach them how to talk.

Children can't learn spoken language without someone teaching them how language works. Parents are the only ones who can do this. No professional can be there to help your child learn how to communicate when they have a bad dream at night. A language facilitator parent does this naturally. The shift in mindset from "Somebody fix my kid" to "I want to do this myself" is what is required of a language facilitator parent.

<u>*Testimonial from a parent who made the shift.*</u>

Marci is our superpower!

My son is close to 3 years old, he used to label well but was not conversational and not make many meaningful sentences till about 3 weeks back.

My son has been a case of Otitis media (middle ear fluid) with recurrent ear infections and speech delay.

We were very worried and started using flash cards and other means to have our child talk. We taught him words and therefore he labelled well with 1-2 words and putting forward his needs either by showing us what he needs or by using 1-2 words.

Since he was not very confident in using natural language, he did not engage much in group activities and had very little participation in his childcare. His childcare said, he is brilliant, but he is not social and that made us worry more.

Our recent pediatrician visit was heart-breaking since my son refused to interact with her, he just completely shut down in front of her and therefore she raised red flags, which made me so fearful and worried that I was scared of taking any speech therapy or seeking any help. The question of 'what if' somebody labels my child came to mind and I didn't know what to do. I knew he is fine and just needed some time and help and I wasn't sure how to help him.

I think connecting with Marci and taking her program was one of the best decisions we made. She heard us and understood our problems, unfortunately not many educated professionals have the time nowadays to listen to parents and what they feel.
Her strategies have helped us, our son is making sentences, not only with us but also with his caretakers...he is engaging in activities in just 3 weeks. It's like magic :).

We know it will take time to get to the next level of conversations and for him to start interacting more with his friends but there is a huge difference in his confidence and his speech and how he asks for things and shops for himself, it feels like a dream come true.

Marci's information on parent's fear and the new language facilitation strategies have made 'us' parents so confident, my mind is at peace, I can focus better with my son and pay more attention to facilitate his language development. I highly recommend Marci and can't thank her enough :). "
~ Shweta (from India, now living with her family in Australia)

Criteria Necessary for a Child to Start Talking Quickly with Language Facilitation

Most late-talking children are excellent candidates for learning natural speech and language from their parents. What I have learned over decades of work as a speech therapist is that no matter what the diagnosis or overall root cause, children do start talking when their parents facilitate language using the right strategies.

In the past 2 years, I have worked with nearly 100 families in 12 different countries. The children are aged from 24 months to 10 years old and their parents reported root cause diagnoses including autism spectrum disorder (ASD), apraxia, ear fluid, prematurity, brain disorders, vision problems, extreme fever diagnosed as a virus, immune disorders, family trauma, and global developmental delay, just to name a few. The truth is, each child who is late talking, has their own unique combination of root causes and blockages that have resulted in their current communication system.

There are only a few, basic criteria to be met for late talkers to learn verbal speech from their parents.

The child must be able to hear speech sounds consistently and that's at 30 decibels or louder.

Children do not need to hear perfectly to talk, however, clear hearing is necessary for clear articulation of speech. If a child is not hearing well due to ear fluid or some other physiological blockage, this root cause must be addressed prior to attempting language facilitation. The child must be able to consistently hear over time to develop their listening skills.

Listening to consistently spoken, clear speech is key so the child can use the rhythm and "song" of the spoken language to help them as they are learning. Children need to hear well to process all the speech sounds in words as others talk to them. If the child's hearing is muffled or blocked, their speech will also be imprecise. Even short periods when hearing falls below 30 decibels can affect speech. Hearing loss due to ear fluid is the most common cause of late-talking I have seen over 30 years of working with children.

<u>The child should have a physically healthy body, and especially the head and neck (ENT) system of ears, nose, mouth and throat.</u>

The child needs to be able to hear as I mentioned, and their sinuses, mouth, and throat must also be healthy. This means the need to be free from recurrent infection, and congestion. Tongue and lip ties (short ligaments in the mouth) and palatal clefts (holes or incomplete palate development) must be resolved. The child must be able to eat the foods that they want to eat via chewing and swallowing. Disruptions in ability to suck from a nipple, eat from a spoon, chew foods, or swallow safely indicate potential neurological issues that require specific evaluation from professionals who do neurological imaging. This is the only way to determine the root causes of the motor disturbances.

Language facilitation will help the child, however if there are significant blockages identified in the neural pathways for mouth movement, there will be issues with speech production. Interventions such as chiropractic, and tDCS stimulation used in combination with language facilitation have shown promise in helping re-develop the damaged pathways via neural plasticity, resulting in true natural spoken language emergence.

* Note* Many late talkers have food sensitivities. Food aversion is not the same as dysphagia, or physical problems with eating. Parents should never force a child to eat food or distract them to get them to eat because this does not address their food aversion.

Eating and talking go together. If it isn't fun to eat, then your late-talking child will develop anxiety surrounding eating. Without language to communicate this, the late-talking child may develop behaviors such as refusing all foods. Aversion to eating often present in late-talking children, especially if they have sensory processing issues. However, food aversion is a choice, not a physiological problem, and many late-talker's parents can teach them to eat a variety of healthy foods safely.

The child must have made some meaningful vocal sounds on their own.

The child may have said words inconsistently or even speech like babbling and lost them, or if a child is nonverbal but they could be using just vowel sounds or screeching. Other children use environmental sounds to imitate actions or characters. If they've made any meaningful kind of vocalizations that may or may not even sound like words, then your child meets the criteria for this. This criterion checks that a child's lungs and "voice box" (their speech producing system) works. Children who are ready to start talking, have figured out that mouth works to make sounds that other people react to.

The child has learned other skills from the parents.

These can be things you have taught them, such as to give you their hand, or it can be things they learned on their own, such as to come to the kitchen to get food when they smell food and see you are cooking. If your child has demonstrated that they can learn other things from you, even by watching you, then you're going to be able to teach them verbal speech.

The child must want to communicate their needs and ideas.

You can see your child wants to communicate by considering how you know what they want now, even though they aren't talking. If they're dragging you around to things, or they're bringing you stuff, or they're yelling, or acting out their messages, these are their current communication system. Most children desperately want to communicate all of their needs, feelings, ideas, and opinions. This is necessary for success with language facilitation, because you can't teach a child to talk if they don't want to communicate with you at all.

The Most Challenging Blockages

Over decades of working with thousands of families, I have identified some characteristics that limit and/or completely block progress. Language facilitation has worked for every family whose child meets the above criteria; however, parents must know that no intervention strategy will work for every family. Some blockages are easy to spot, however challenging to address without the assistance of a professional who can facilitate change at the neurological level. This means that the targeted intervention must somehow directly affect change in the brain that will trigger neural plasticity.

Children who rarely (less than 20% of waking time) initiate interaction with their parents will not be able to learn language naturally from them.

This would be an indication of a very low cognitive level and is present only in a very small percentage of children. These children don't try to interact with you at all and never try to request things. The only time that they'll communicate or interact with others is when they are being cared for.

Unresolved seizures cause ongoing cognitive damage.

Children with this level of damage to the neurological system require direct brain stimulation combined with language facilitation to potentially trigger neural plasticity.

If the child is physically unwell and inconsolable more than twice a day for whatever reason on a consistent basis, their energy is too focused on their physical needs to learn language effectively. Oral motor or movement problems that are going to prohibit verbal speech, are identified in children who cannot independently coordinate their mouth to eat or drink.

If a child is on non-oral feeding due to throat or swallowing problems and the child is able to make sounds with their mouth, then they can become verbal. It's the children who can't live without assistance to eat, dress themselves, or move from place to place who require more assistance or an alternative, nonverbal communication system due to inability to interact outside of general recognition.

One of the reasons for this is that language facilitation takes conscious effort from parents. If the child needs help to get through every aspect of their life for basic survival, then facilitating verbal speech may not be something that parents can manage on top of all those other daily problem-solving things that you have to do.

For language facilitation to be successful, the child must have some basic attention to be interested in SOMETHING. Even nonverbal kids have patterns of behavior that indicate their preferences and parents can usually spot them. If a child is never interested in anything ever then parents will be challenged to find opportunities to facilitate language. When a child is unable to learn any basic tasks, even with demonstration, they will be challenged to learn language naturally.

These are the children who are not reaching to you when you go to pick them up. They are not able to learn to hold your hand (you always must grab theirs) or follow you when you lead them. If the child is unable to produce any speech sounds during their independent play, when they're doing things on their own, or when they're doing the things that they love the most, then they will be challenged to learn verbal speech.

If your child is not making any noises and they are completely silent all the time except for screaming and crying, even when they are the happiest, language facilitation is going to be a challenge. If your child does display any of these other warning signs, then you need to discuss those things with your child's healthcare practitioner.

In 3 decades of practice as a speech pathologist I have only encountered only two interventions that result in any significant spontaneous spoken language development in late talking children who demonstrate obvious neurological signs. They are chiropractic intervention for neck alignment adjustment and transcranial direct current stimulation (tDCS). Information supporting biomedical interventions to improve brain function are also showing promise, however in my experience, the results are highly variable. Parents are encouraged to investigate these modalities if your child is showing significant cognitive and/or motor disturbances that are affecting your child's ability to eat and/or talk. The most important thing to remember is that even with the best physical intervention to address brain function, without language facilitation from parents to retrain the language learning parts of the brain, the child will not learn to develop natural language.

Indicators of Excellent Prognosis for Development of Verbal Speech
Fast

These are the characteristics displayed by kids who talk FAST, many even within the first week, like Shweta's son. One very common pattern I have observed over 3 decades of speech pathology work is that late talkers who are amazing at problem solving always talk fast. These are the kids who are great at communicating without using words. Most of them have made up their own "language". They're often great at pantomiming or acting out everything, and they have great facial expressions. These are children who have been spoken to a lot, and/or have heard a lot of speech on videos. These late talkers are typically visual communicators and while they already have a ton of language already inside of them and know a lot of words, they don't know how to access and use them. They're just waiting for you to unlock it.

If your child is great at communicating their messages with you with actions, you are probably great at guessing what they are communicating by watching them. These kids are super great at learning words, because they quickly figure out that words are a lot easier than acting out all their messages. These brilliant problem-solvers are the kids that can figure out locks, climb up cabinets, and get around any obstacle. No matter where you hide something, if they want it, they find it.

The kids who start talking fast, are also the kids who are experts with technology. These are the children who learn how to search and watch videos in different languages and use multiple different applications. These tasks require a child to learn the rules of the systems and work within the rules to get their desired outcome. It's amazing problem-solving training. Those kids who are amazing with problem solving, respond so well to the language facilitation process, because it is a problem-solving approach to learning language.

You, as the parents, can easily figure out what's going on with your child and what they are trying to communicate. If you show them how to use words instead of their own behavior "language" it makes communication easier, for them. They don't have to act out every message. You will show your child that all they must do is use the words they already know, and you will show them exactly how to use them via your demonstration. Then they make progress really fast.

Another criterion that really shows excellent prognosis is when kids are strong-willed and love to learn things on their own terms. These kids know what they do, and they like to know how they do it. They are usually quite bossy too. These super-smart late talkers are very controlling, and they may also be perfectionists. They do whatever they love to do over and over until they get it perfect. They also can switch gears in a heartbeat and move on to the next challenge. These kids learn and process things internally.

Some late-talkers think and learn so fast that they can't share their ideas with speech, so parents often get stuck over teaching and asking kids to say words that they already know, which can end up in frustration for both parents and kids.

Even though being strong-willed, controlling, and a perfectionist sounds like it might present a problem, this characteristic is a sign of strong intelligence and fast learning. Once you help your strong-willed child embark on a language learning mission, they put all that effort into learning how to use the words they know and get better and better and better at talking fast.

Most kids have some of these strong-willed characteristics. It's their internal protection system. In fact, when you think about it, most children have little regard for new ideas. Until they're convinced that the activity will be fun, they are skeptical. Parents learn that when they need to present a new idea, that they need to explain the situation in terms the child can understand and somehow get the child interested. Once this happens, the child will happily have fun and participate with your help.

Consider the child who tries to eat ice cream for the first time. The parent knows that the child has never had something so cold in their mouth. So first the parents give a small taste and wait for a reaction. At first, the child is surprised and may even react negatively to the cold. When the parent encourages the child to focus on the yummy taste and shows the child how fun it is to lick the sweet cream, then the child's reaction changes. The parent has helped the child experience this new idea and change their mind! Now they want ice cream all the time.

Strong-willed kids learn the things they are interested in FAST because they don't like being "schooled". It's like a double-edged sword. They do learn fast, but they also want to manipulate and control their environment - including their parents. They're real bossy. They spend a lot of effort "telling" parents what to do even non-verbally. They're pushing everyone around.

Strong-willed late-talkers need to keep the illusion of control because it is their comfort-zone and communication survival system. They KNOW that they are not good at using words, but they always want to be in charge. These kiddos are so smart, that they have learned how to problem-solve every situation to try to AVOID talking at all costs. They get whatever they want with the least amount of effort. They put the responsibility on everyone else to guess what they want and try to read their mind.

Many late talkers refuse to try say words because they are perfectionists and they don't want to get it wrong. So, they've trained everyone to try to guess. It's what I call the never-ending game of charades.

I always tell parents, to be aware that, once they learn how to use the words they know, the strong-willed late talkers are going to start ordering parents around verbally! With language facilitation, we teach children the words THEY want to say. So, if your late talker is literally pushing you around with their hands now to communicate, they're going to start verbally pushing you around too!

If you believe your child is a late talker who doesn't display any of those most challenging blockages, then you can certainly breathe a sigh of relief, because your child definitely has the same potential to develop natural speech as his or her talkative peers, no matter what has caused their late talking.

I have seen language facilitation work for thousands of kids with all different kinds of physical root causes for the late-talking and it always works, if the family meet those positive criteria. If your child is making some sounds and is a good problem-solver, then it's very highly likely that your child's going to start to talk quickly when you do the right kind of intervention.

The Secrets for Language Facilitation Success

#1. If it isn't FUN, it ISN'T fun.

Your strategies and language facilitation opportunities must be FUN, and it must be fun for both the kids and the parents. Because, if the tasks are just another chore to add to your already long list, you're not going to want to do them, and you are certainly not going to enjoy them. If you want verbal speech to be the main form of communication in your household, then everything surrounding talking must be fun for both you and your child. You must eliminate every speech and language facilitation strategy, intervention, class, therapist, or circumstance that is not easy, happy, safe, or FUN for your child and your family. If your child is crying or screaming through therapy, it's not helping them learn anything at all and causing repeated traumatic experiences that very commonly result in anxiety. This book will provide you with the process to systematically adopt the habits of a language facilitator and teach your child how to naturally develop and use all of verbal speech that is inside of them with FUN.

#2. Parents Must Take Responsibility.

You as parents must take responsibility for not just what is going on as you move forward, but how things got to be where they are right now. The actions that you have taken so far have contributed to cause the current circumstances of your child's language development. You cannot change what you have done in the past, however you can make conscious choices to do the right things moving forward. If you find yourself slipping into habits that are not consciously focused on your path forward, then you are wasting your time.

#3. Language Facilitation Must Happen During Everyday Activities.

To really make language facilitation of natural speech and language work, it has to be centered around the family activities and experiences that you do every day. Language facilitation must happen every day as often as possible. You must practice your strategies frequently in order to help change your habits. It's a lifestyle, long-term, fundamental change in how your family communicates. This is key to change your family's nonverbal communication habits and shift from the nonverbal language systems you are using into spoken language. You are going to start to help your child shift whatever they are already using now for communication into verbal speech.

#4. Language Facilitation is a Lifetime Journey.

Parents often come to this journey with expectations of "measurable progress" such as timeframes, numbers of words said, or specific skills like answering questions. Children all develop spoken language at their own pace. Language facilitation is not something you "try for a few weeks to see what happens." If parents compare their children to others development instead of keeping them in line with the child's pace, this will result in frustration for both the child and the parents. The parents and they abandon their new habits and fall back into old prompting strategies just to hear kids say words.

Your worry mindset will try to sneak in and block you. It happens to everybody. Even my most successful language facilitator parents tell me that they find themselves wanting to slip back into the wrong habits such as prompting, even though they know it is not helping their child. This happens when parents try to push their late talkers through the process of speech development faster than they are ready because somehow, they were triggered to compare their child with other children. When this happens, parents worry about their child's lack of speech and all their focus shifts away from having fun with the process to fear and worry about the future. The current, effective language facilitation habits that take more time get abandoned for desperation prompting so the parent can feel better hearing a few words. Children perceive their parent's desperation energy and recoil from the increased demands. You must take responsibility for consciously focusing your thoughts and efforts on your everyday process. You must TRUST that your child is capable of spoken language and that you are the key to helping them find the words that you know are inside. It's important to consistently analyze your mindset as an ongoing process if you want to see long-lasting change.

What is Really Going On

Why is my child late talking? This is the question that keeps most parents up at night. When I ask parents what they believe is causing their child's language delay, they try to answer this question by using a diagnosis. I hear "My child is not talking because he has ____". If you want to get a comprehensive diagnosis you should schedule an appointment with a certified speech-language pathologist. There are many diagnoses given to children who are late talking but, none of them matter because they don't give parents the answer to the question... WHY?

If you don't identify exactly what's going on to block your child's natural spoken language development and why the blockage is happening, you're not going to be able to eliminate it. That's why it's very important that you consciously analyze your family communication strategies, methods, and habits. Honest, self-analysis can be your best tool to identify and eliminate all spoken language blockages throughout your lifetime language facilitation process.

To help you figure out what is going on, first, I will describe the progression of natural speech and language development. This information will help you know where your child is right now along the natural language development process.

I will also describe the process that has worked for families all over the world to help their late-talking child overcome their resistance to saying words and shift from nonverbal communication habits and patterns to wanting to learn how to use natural spoken language.

To help you visualize the process, I have shared a complete case study detailing the process of one family's first year with language facilitation. You will learn how this family, and all of the others in our Waves of Communication Community have helped their children shift from late talkers to chatterboxes.

The Progression of Speech and Language Development

Natural speech and language progression kind of goes like a snowball. It starts in infancy with very little responsibility for independent expression. From their first day of life, babies start to learn how communication works. They learn very quickly that when they consciously do certain behaviors, they get certain responses. As they grow up, their needs, wants, and ideas become more complex. So, their behaviors become more and more specific and complex to help their parents guess and respond to exactly what they want. This is how late talkers develop their complex nonverbal communication "language". Children always start their language development using behaviors designed to help others guess what they want. They need to use behaviors first because they haven't heard enough actual talking to learn words until they are at least 9-10 months old. This is the earliest time when children start to try to "say" things to communicate.

As children get older, they have more interest in sharing their experiences with others, so they start to imitate the things their parents do and say. After children start to understand words, they take a little bit more responsibility to listen and learn from others as well as to communicate their ideas. It becomes increasingly important to children, as they develop their own ideas and personalities, that they make sure their parents understand all the child's unique ideas. When children are engaged in an activity with their parents, they listen when parents talk about the things that they are doing. This is how children learn spoken language naturally; by listening to the words their parents are saying.

Phase #1 – Exploring spoken words for usefulness and fun

Children move through phases along their spoken language development journey, each building on the other. The first phase emerges in typically developing language by 18 months. At this phase, children are using only a handful of words. The words may be inaccurate and overgeneralized, so for example, they might be calling every animal a dog. Words may come and go, with 2 or 3 of them typically used consistently to label or request their favorite things such as Kitty or drink or Mom. At this phase, the child is talking for the purposes of getting someone's attention, indicating needs, and having fun listening to themselves talk. The reason for them to be saying words is usually very self-centered and self-focused. There are usually few verbs and the communications are needs-based.

The sounds that they're saying are just emerging and may be inconsistent at the beginning. All the words may sound similar and words may be mixed in with babbling. In this phase, children may say words different ways at different times because they're just learning. The child's speech sounds are highly related to their hearing, so if any history is ear fluid is in your child's history, there is a good chance sounds may not be clear, especially at first.

Receptive language in the exploring language phase is always much better functionally than expressive language. Even in phase one of spoken language development, children are already understanding and following 1-2 step directions such as "come here" or "give Daddy a kiss". They understand a lot of words, however, especially very young children, must rely on visual cues to understand every message. They also need to hear a lot of spoken language models to help them grow their vocabulary and learn how to use the words functionally.

This is the phase when children who want to talk are in active vocabulary-building mode, so they very often like to watch, listen to, and do their favorite things over and over and over. This is how Children memorize the words they know. Whatever they are focusing their attention on at this phase is where they are hearing language models and forming their first vocabulary.

It is common when children first start talking, that they only say words only to themselves, for their own entertainment. Many children memorize words from listening to their favorite videos, songs, and rhymes over and over. They memorize words and phrases that they hear people around them saying frequently. At all stages of spoken language development, even though adulthood, people need to spend time practicing the words and phrases that we have memorized.

When they are alone, kids think about their favorite things. They replay the memories in their mind, and practice saying their favorite words out loud. Many children say their first words when they are alone in their bed before sleeping or when they first wake up. Children use the time when they are alone to practice saying their favorite words over and over so they can figure out for themselves how to use their words later when they want to share their fun messages with you.

Phase #2 – Harnessing the power of speech

The next phase of speech development usually hits around 24 months old because at this age, kids are exposed to new experiences every day. The learning curve at this age can be very steep if there is a lot of change or activity in the child's life. This is the age when many kids experience common childhood illness which can block the whole process. Typically developing language grows rapidly at this stage from just a few inconsistent words to children using 2-3-word phrases that express their basic needs with more detail because they have more vocabulary. For example, they can now ask for the "blue cup", want to take a "small bite" or be able to tell you "no eat". At this phase children always label their favorite things, usually combined with wanting to physically touch them and explore with all their physical senses.

Another more advanced skill at this phase is children learn new words all the time in the context of sharing their experiences with other people. At this phase, children should be saying things like, "Me Go bye-bye", "my cookie", or "Love you," because they have experienced the opportunity to hear parents use these phrases in all different contexts. Many children can label a few colors, letters and numbers. At this age, children will make a lot of mistakes with their verbal speech because they are learning so fast.

Speech clarity, 24 months, should be understandable by most people with some developmental articulation errors. Their speech will sound cute.

As far apart as receptive and expressive language are in the first phase, in phase two, the gap is often even wider. Children should be able to easily understand and follow 2 to 3 step directions and complex sentences, however they may be independently getting what they want because they are also developing their problem-solving and independence skills. Children at this phase are more interested in making other people understand them than they are in focusing on the specifics of the speech they are hearing; this is why they can understand so much more than they can say. They don't often pay close enough attention to the individual words, because they are more focused on exploring their world.

This level of speech comes with confidence that helps children develop more independence and try to communicate socially with others. When the speech is clear and slow enough, and when they're in a good mood, children at this phase should be able to follow a basic storyline when you read a book to them, especially if they have heard the story before.

Phase #3 – The Wannabe Confident Talker

As kids enter the next phase, typically at about 30 months, they make another big jump in spoken language development. In this phase, children should be independently telling little stories, using 5-to-7-word sentences. Their speech should be well past basic needs and include lots of verbs, adjectives, and prepositions. They need this level of speech to be able to direct others, (become bossy). In this phase, children have full speech confidence and they will say new words out loud all the time even if they are not correct.

Children develop the ability to talk about the things that they are thinking about. They will begin to talk about their events out of sight, such as how their sibling took their toy, or a child had a birthday party at preschool. They'll remember names of their friends and their teachers, even if they can't say them well. In this phase, vocabulary words will continue to increase in both number and complexity and there'll be more and more novel ideas coming out all the time. Kids in this phase are usually very egotistical and when their speech becomes confident, they often start ordering other people around with more passion and more specific directions as well.

In this phase, the child's speech may be the hardest for people to understand. The child is not skilled at talking yet and may try to use fast speech and longer sentences than they are ready for. Their minds are full of all the new learning and their expressive vocabulary is rapidly trying to keep up with their comprehension.

They are usually moving around a lot at this phase with newly developing motor skills like running climbing and kicking balls and not paying attention to speaking clearly. So, overall talking at this phase is harder for everyone to understand, this is true especially with people who are not familiar to the child. At this age, Kids don't typically like to try to "fix" their speech so others can understand them more easily. They don't have time! They are too busy learning new things and trying to find the words they need to communicate their next message to worry about saying it with all the right sounds in all the right places. Children who are confident talkers expect everyone to know what they are saying, because in their mind, they have communicated it perfectly, even when it sounds exactly like every other word they have said.

Children who have the opportunity to hear good language models every day, usually become more and more motivated to try harder to talk as they see the effect their speech has on the people around them. They try very hard to make sure other people understand their messages exactly. This is why the confident talkers quickly develop speech and move through this phase in less than 6 months.

Phase #4 – The Confident Chatterbox

The last phase - when language becomes complex, usually comes at around 36 months. In this phase, kids should be using conversation, exchanging new and thoughtful ideas, sharing their opinions. This is the stage when children are starting to understand jokes and use their own intentional humor. Kids can now verbally challenge other people's ideas and start to negotiate. They have an insatiable desire to learn the words for the ideas in their minds and they independently try hard to clearly express their ideas. They confidently share their independent ideas and they also share their feelings verbally. They can go on and on for hours when they are talking about the things they love.

In this stage, almost everybody should be able to understand their speech. The child's speech typically will get increasingly clearer and more intelligible with practice. The child may have a few noticeable articulation errors with certain words; however, these things correct when the child hears the words spoken slowly and clearly, and then tries hard to use accurate pronunciation. There might be some habits that make a child's speech sound cute, but they will fade with maturity.

As far as comprehension, the child should be able to memorize longer phrases such as lines in songs, and retell stories they have heard, especially their favorite ones. Expressive language has caught up with their receptive language. Children can understand details in new stories when you read them and retell the same stories with their own twist. They develop their personality and communicate their preferences at the chatterbox phase. In fact, a favorite topic for a chatterbox is to critique the things they experience and share their opinions with others. Children easily remember things that happened before, especially emotionally charged experiences. They notice and share their opinions about "drama". They remember promises made to them as well and expect people to keep their promises!

This progression of spoken language development the same for all children who learn their first language. Typically, children move through the phases within a few months of the milestones I reported, however, every child moves through these phases at their own pace. Some children are using sentences at 18 months, others don't talk until 4 years and they are both totally normal. The speed of progress through the phases depends on the child's language learning skills and opportunity to practice.

Skills Necessary for Natural Spoken Language Development
1. Ability to self-regulate emotions and process sensory input without fear
2. Consistently hear, attend to, and focus on parents and caregivers clearly spoken words
3. Move freely to explore and experience new things to talk about
4. Listen to and focus on their parents talking
5. See their parents' mouths while they are talking

These are the only skills a child needs to be able to learn spoken language from their parents. Any disruption in these five experiences will cause a child to be late talking. If your child who hasn't met these milestone guidelines, then they are a late talker. Something has blocked their language learning experiences and spoken expressive language development stopped. Instead of moving forward in their communication by learning spoken language, the late-talking child remains stuck in their never-ending job of creating a nonverbal communication "language" so parents can understand their needs and ideas. As the late-talking child learns new things and develops their own preferences and novel ideas, they must create more and more intricate ways to nonverbally share their messages with others.

I believe every nonverbal child is a late talker. Something has happened to limit the necessary experiences for spoken language development and hold up their expressive communication. When that happens, the child leaves the blocked spoken language path. They became a nonverbal communicator instead of a talker out of necessity. I have observed in thousands of cases, that once the blockages are identified, and resolved, then kids get back on the spoken language path and they learn to speak naturally.

Self-Analysis – How to figure out what is really going on

What parents really need to know is the actual root cause of their child's speech development blockages. You need to look beyond the diagnosis label to identify and address any physiological root cause for blockage in the child's hearing, vision, attention, or movement before you can expect your child to learn language naturally. A diagnosis without understanding the physical root cause is incomplete. Comprehensive evaluation of all your child's physical health systems is necessary until you find the problem that caused delayed development of one or more of the following: hearing/listening, vision/seeing, mouth movement/eating, breathing/lung support, walking/getting around. When any of these basic functions are blocked, spoken language cannot develop. These physical "systems" must be consistently healthy and functional for a child to be successful developing verbal speech ongoing. If any of these systems are even temporarily disabled, the child will seek alternative (nonspeech) forms of communication and get off the spoken language development path.

While the physiological blockage may be the root of your child's late talking, you can't stop your investigation and intervention with the physical body. There is a lot more to understanding the cause of late talking than physical blockages. Children who have had some physical blockage to speech learning have necessarily had to develop an alternative way to communicate. Even children who are completely healthy may be late-talking due to environmental influences. Parents must consider all the situations, behaviors, habits and patterns in your child's life that have contributed to the way your child is communicating right now. Some children become very controlling in their attempts to teach parents how to understand their behaviors. This can make them resistant to parents trying to teach them a new way to talk.

Nonverbal children learn to communicate through their physical behaviors. All their behaviors that seem directed toward others are designed to help another person understand and respond to their messages. Late-talkers develop their nonverbal communication behaviors with their own problem-solving and trial and error. They try behaviors over and over to learn what behaviors get their parents attention and makes sure parents understand their feelings. Late-talking kids pay attention to how parents respond to them and learn when to use the right behavior to get whatever they need with the least amount of effort. When a parent tries to change a late-talking child's primary communication system by force, it usually results in power-struggles characterized by resistance, anxiety, and frustration on the part of the parent and the child.

To learn anything new, children need to feel happy and safe. They need to receive consistent, positive encouragement toward independent learning and problem-solving. Children need to be free from anxiety and fear and feel comfortable listening to adults and children talking naturally while they learn about life. They need to be encouraged to move around freely and explore their environment on their terms with appropriate boundaries to keep them safe. When natural, independent learning opportunities are restricted, negative feelings arise that further block a late-talker's interest in learning spoken language, even after they are completely healthy.

Parents are easily able to perceive feelings of anxiety, fear, worry, anger, and frustration in their late-talking child, especially when the resulting behaviors happen frequently. You must intuitively analyze all possible circumstances to identify what could have triggered these consistent negative emotions in your child. This is how you identify the emotional root cause for the behaviors and the root cause of your child's late talking. You analyze your everyday experiences to identify the situations and habits that are continuing to affect your child. Then, you can be on your way deciding what changes need to be made in your child's life to eliminate these negative feelings and taking the right action toward progress.

You have also made a commitment to help your child learn to talk the right way and I want to help you get yourself organized from the very beginning.

Holistically Analyze Your Family Communication System

You must analyze your child's current communication methods so that you can understand exactly what specific verbal and nonverbal systems they have developed to communicate right now. You also need to closely to look at your own part in the process including how you are responding to their communication behaviors. You need to self-evaluate your own communication with your child. The way that you speak and the words that you use are the models for the speech that your child is developing. Your child is always watching and listening to you to learn language. Your language models need to represent the speech that you want to hear.

You need to analyze your child's habitual language/word learning methods so you can use their favorite methods to teach them. How did your child learn to understand you? What did you do to help them? Where did your child learn to say the words they do say now? How do they use that speech functionally with you? Identify which of your current language facilitation methods are working to help your child listen and focus on your carefully spoken language. Alternatively, realize there are habits you are using every day that could be blocking your child's language learning experiences and consciously try to eliminate these habits.

All the information and awareness you will gain from your analysis will help you create your new language facilitation plan to move forward using only communication methods and language facilitation strategies that focus on the path toward natural language learning.
Analyze Your Mindset Every Day

The late-talker's mindset is really important in the process of natural language learning. You remember I wrote about how children need confidence to spark their interest in trying to use the words they have memorized. Mindset issues such as anxiety, worry, and fear directly affect a child's willingness to participate in even the most fun learning opportunities. Your child may be experiencing these mindset blocks that are keeping them stuck in nonverbal communication.

Parent mindset is equally as important to facilitate natural language learning. Parents who remain focused on their own anxiety, worry, and fear are distracted from offering the right natural speech learning experiences. Because parents naturally have an intuitive connection with their kids, children also perceive how their parents are feeling. You will need to analyze your mindset as well as the mindset of all persons in the child's life, including their attitudes about the child's health issues, developmental delays, and behaviors. Your mindset and attitude toward these things directly affect your behavior and ability to help your child in the way that they need.

You need to determine and release what is fueling your negative emotions of anxiety, worry, or fear. It is normal to have these feelings as a parent and it shows your extreme love for your child. However, you must understand that these feelings are blocking your child's progress and accept your responsibility to change. Nobody can change your feelings and actions except you.

The results of your analysis will provide you with all the information that you need to eliminate blockages from your child's language learning experience, to the best of your ability. Every family is different, and you are going to need to honestly analyze your own situation to find the answers you're looking for. I will guide you through the process in this book, however, you are on your own to make the changes necessary to see a different outcome.

Remember, parents are the most powerful influence in every child's spoken language development. Both positive and negative influences, even subconscious ones caused by internal fears, have significant effect on the entire process.

It's important for parents to become conscious and consistent with self-analysis, because you will be doing it ongoing for the rest of your child's life. Consistent, ongoing analysis is necessary, even after you eliminate massive blockages. This is because change creates the unknown. As your family moves through everyday life together, new external and internal blockages will constantly pop up. That's life! When you are checking in with conscious and honest analysis about your current experiences it is easy to spot the blockages.

I will guide you through the process, so you can practice and become proficient. This way, you will have the tools you need to turn things around again when you find yourself feeling stuck in the future at any point in your language facilitation journey - and you will. You can always see a bump in progress when you go back to self-analysis and eliminate any mindset blocks that have wiggled their way into your everyday habits.

Helping Your Child Overcome Resistance to Talking

There is a 5-step process for helping late talkers shift from nonverbal communication patterns to natural spoken language. This process has been the foundation for every language facilitation plan I have created in my Waves of Communication custom coaching program that has helped every family find success. It is my proven process to help parents teach their children how to use the words they need to share their wisdom with the world. This simple process turns parents into language facilitators and children into talkers.

Step #1 – Eliminate Physical Root Causes.

Any physiological issues that cause chronic discomfort must be resolved so that the child can meet the criteria for verbal speech. The child must be physically able to engage, listen, and move their mouth when they want to. They need well enough to have a clear view of people's faces.

Step #2 – Adopt the Mindset of a Language Facilitator.

You must trust the process and eliminate your expectations and comparisons. Eliminate your fears and worry to focus your energy on strategies you know will help you. Most importantly, parents must be prepared to encourage and allow your child to develop speech naturally at their own pace without judgement.

Step #3 – If it isn't FUN, it ISN'T fun

Eliminate any situations, habits, behaviors, or strategies that consistently cause negative feelings for you or your child. Prompting and exchange-based methods that you might be using must be replaced with language opportunities that are easy, happy, safe, and fun.

Parents must limit therapies that utilize exchange based or reward-based systems. Therapists always need to use prompting to do their therapy intervention in the structured therapy session. While you can control prompting in your home, you don't have any say over how much prompting your child receives when they are in therapy. It is advisable to avoid interventions that utilize behavior training, repetition, repeated prompting, reinforcements, and exchange-based modalities.

Therapy approaches that assist parents with language facilitation focus on child-directed activities, social-interaction philosophies, and relationship-based intervention. Developmental and play-based language approaches are closer to language facilitation strategies. Therapy sessions should always include parent involvement. Parent coaching time should be prioritized instead of an afterthought. Therapist and parents can help late-talkers progress faster when you share your effective strategies. Parents are responsible for communication with therapists, asking questions to receive guidance, and following up with the strategies between sessions.

Therapists have very little power over long-term speech and language development via inconsistent 30-60-minute sessions. Wise parents use their therapists as resources to help them facilitate language every day.

Step #4 - Help your children feel safe making big changes.

Your job is to help your late-talking child (who probably doesn't like talking) to believe that speech is easy. The only way to help a child shift from current communication habits is to make talking seem very attractive and easy to try. You will need to help your late talker WANT to shift away from the non-verbal language that they've been using their whole life and use something new as their go to communication. In order to do this, you must always help your child succeed.

Children learn by watching and listening to their parents. They try things when you encourage them and make it fun. Think about how you have encouraged your child to try something new that is fun. It's easy to help your child overcome fear and change their mindset when they have a small, successful, enjoyable experience such as tasting ice cream for the first time or jumping on a big trampoline. Speech can be easy and fun when you play with sounds and words while making silly faces in a mirror, make animal and vehicle noises, sing songs, or change your voice to like your child's favorite character.

If your child struggles to say words, tell them that you know it is hard. Remind them that you are not in a hurry to push any outcome and that you appreciate every attempt. Empower them to keep trying by reminding them how much you love their speech and that you think every attempt at talking is perfect. Because, it doesn't matter if the speech is not accurate, the attempt is what you are encouraging. Parents should celebrate every effort your child makes to explore talking as a new way of communicating. Your child will learn that you are there to help them try at things they believe are challenging and their success will show them that their "work" is worth the effort. Once late-talkers learn the basics of how words work from their parents, they quickly learn to use you as a resource to learn the words for their favorite things. This way they can ask for them more easily.

Step #5 - Empower your child to adopt the mindset of a confident independent talker.

To make the shift, your child needs to own verbal speech as their new go to communication method for all their communication messages. It is easy for children to learn to use words to get things, however, communication of their unique ideas and emotions is a different level of language. Conversational language requires a child to independently form verbal messages to represent the pictures they have in their mind.

When the late-talking child has figured out how to learn language from parents, they then learn how to watch and listen to the other people in their environment to see how they use speech and language to communicate too. The late talker then tries to say the words they learned from listening to everyone and share their own messages. Usually, people respond in a very positive way by understanding the child's messages and praising them for trying to talk. The late talker experiences the ease and functionality of talking and this helps them shift their mindset to choosing the easier option. With practice, the late talker understands how much more effective, useful, and FUN it is to share their ideas with words and how much easier it is for people to understand them when they talk.

All the gateways to spoken language development are open at this point and the child starts to actively learn more words and practice talking more frequently. With all this conscious effort, the child's spoken language ability continually improves. This is how confident independent spoken language emerges naturally, at the child's pace. Parents have empowered their late-talking children to share their messages independently and actively learn language naturally from everyone and the learning never stops. Late-talkers become talkers and stop relying on parents to interpret their non-verbal behaviors.

Language Facilitation Case Study - The story of G

I am sharing the following case study as an example of how one family moved through the process of helping their withdrawn late-talking child shift from nonverbal communication patterns into the kid who makes everybody's friend. As you read through the description of their experiences,

I suggest you consider how this family moved through the process of understanding the blockages in their child's environment and taking action to eliminate them. Perhaps, you will be able to use their experiences to help you analyze your own situation.

The first language facilitation case study is about 7.5-year-old G. The information for their story has been provided as a report from his mother.

G's Mom is from China, his Dad is American, and they live in the United States. Mom reported that there are many men in her family who did not talk until 3 or 4 years old, so G's parents were not concerned about his late talking when the doctor noted he was not saying any words at his 24-month health check. G enjoyed spending time with his parents and followed them around a lot and was also able to play alone well. He is an only child. Between ages 3-6, G lived with his grandmother who cared for him. She spoke Chinese all day and G reportedly could understand her; however, he did not talk. Grandma reportedly anticipated G's needs a lot because he was nonverbal. So, G did not have much practice asking for things like food. He watched a lot of TV and videos and spent a lot of time alone.

At his 3-year pediatrician visit, G was still not talking. The pediatrician referred them for speech therapy and further evaluation with a developmental pediatrician. G was diagnosed with speech delay by the speech therapist and received therapy at a clinic for 6 months, while parents waited for an appointment with a developmental pediatrician. After 6 months of therapy, G didn't talk.

In the developmental evaluation, G did not want to interact with the evaluators, however, he did like to play with the toys on his own and he did interact with his parents in the room. His parents reported that he regularly plays and interacts with them at home the only other symptoms they observed was lining things up. G was diagnosed with mild autism.

Parents initially began sending G to a private preschool with more emphasis on speech and communication with speech therapy provided at the school 3 times per week. G said his first word at 5 years old. After 2 years of therapy and preschool, at 5.5 years old, G was reportedly using a handful of single words to request and label the things that he wanted most, but he never said words on his own. His mom was able to get him to imitate the few words he knew words at home, but only when she used reward.

After 2 years of this preschool, G started to show a change in his behavior. His limited language had caused him to develop a lot of behaviors to communicate. G figured out how to use behaviors to avoid the structured activities at school and his mother's attempts to teach him at home. G frequently threw things, ran away, and destroyed the educational materials. G didn't participate in the group or interact with other children and he required assistance for getting through structured tasks. He was also an elopement risk, because he learned how to open every door both at school and at home.

Alternatively, G learned how to use sweet behavior such as kisses, hugs, or sharing his food or toys to get his parents and teachers to give him affection and stop yelling at him. This change in behavior was reported by teachers to be G's way to avoid structured work. The teachers and therapists started using a reward system with food and toys to help G stay with the class and participate in the activities. Parents did the same at home to limit behaviors and get through activities.

G was also using avoidance behaviors at home. His mom reported that it was increasingly difficult to get G to respond to any people or use any words unless he really wanted something. G's Mom reported feeling even more frustrated and desperate because it was increasingly difficult to take him places in public. G's Mom reported that during this time he would spontaneously erupt into meltdowns with screaming and crying for some small issue, or without any warning at all. She also reported problems with G having no interest in responding to her directions or even to his name. He always wanted to run and touch everything and if she restrained him, he screamed.

At that point, G's parents were guided to begin Applied Behavior Analysis Therapy (ABA) 20 hours per week to focus on the behaviors. The first year, G reportedly made "great strides" in following directions. G reportedly started responding to his parents when they used the prompts and rewards at home as well. G's parents were reportedly happy that he had learned to respond to directions better, however, their primary goals for G have always been spoken language. When G's parents brought their concerns to the ABA therapy provider, they were advised to increase the ABA to 40 hours a week, including daily home visits. This increase in time was reportedly necessary, so therapists could work on communication goals in addition to behavior goals. She also continued private speech therapy weekly to focus on speech.

The communication goals for both ABA and speech therapy focused on teaching G to grab or touch pictures of animals, colors, and many household objects and foods when named. For expressive communication of wants and needs, the therapists used the Picture Exchange Communication System (PECS) to teach G exchange one of the pictures he learned for the object or action that he wanted. G reportedly learned this system quickly and he was given a tablet-based picture system to use at ABA therapy and at home as well. G's parents were reportedly trained to use the system and expected to help G use the tablet to make requests at home and in the community.

Unfortunately, that was when G's parents hit the most common external blockage that faces a LOT of parents in this situation. - They were literally shut down by the very therapists they were paying to help their child. After eliminating all spoken language facilitation, and ignoring their son's anxiety and resistance to the intervention, G's ABA team reportedly told his parents that he is more severe than previously evaluated, and subsequently by a neurologist and 2 other speech therapists that G is not "wired for spoken words" and that he would likely never talk naturally.

G's mom refused to give up and doubled down on her efforts to get G to say spoken words at home. She prompted, begged, held objects out of reach, hid things and asked questions all day long so G would have to use his words. G reportedly was very "strong-willed" and consistently resisted her efforts. He learned how to get everything himself instead of asking. G's Mom learned to use the tablet picture system as instructed by the ABA therapists to avoid behaviors, however, she found the system inconvenient and limiting. That's why she increased her own efforts to prompting him to say words, and started looking into different online programs, systems, and remedies to help her find her son's spoken language.

External blockages continued from the interventionists. G's mother's repeated attempts to get speech pathologists and BCBA to focus goals on verbal speech were met with "data" to show G's amazing "progress" using the communication device. G's parents are both college-educated professionals, and they were provided with data from evidence-based research to reinforce the opinion of the therapy center that children as old as G need to use alternative augmentative communication to be successful.

After a year of full-time ABA, G had started to use more significant avoidance behaviors at home and especially during ABA sessions. At this point, G was 7.5 years old and he was showing daily signs of anger and anxiety. G displayed 20-40-minute meltdowns with screaming and throwing himself on the floor, poop-smearing, throwing and hitting things. G even punched a hole in a wall. Instead of helping G move forward and learn new things, therapists and parents focused their energy on management of these behaviors.

Something even more significant started happening that led to complete blockage of spoken language learning. G slowly and completely lost his interest in listening to people talking, and instead, focused his attention on tablet videos and games. He avoided people and he avoided saying words at all costs. At this point, G was 7.5 years old. He reportedly was able to say about 150 words, however, he only spoke when he was prompted. Additionally, the words were rarely clearly spoken. G typically only said part of the word using a very soft voice. G's Mom reported that he appeared to have no confidence in his speech. She noticed that when she asked him to try to talk, she lost eye contact and he usually walked away. G's mom also reported that his interest in interaction with others decreased and his behavior and anxiety were getting worse. She could see that G was visibly upset by the intervention and the pressure because he frequently whined, cried, and ultimately yelled at everyone instead of talking.

G's mom reported feeling disempowered when therapists told her to ignore the tantrums. She was told "do not comfort G" and "walk away" when he had a meltdown. G's Mom remembers therapists asking her to leave the room when they were in the house, because G always wanted her to console him.

This likely happened, because outside of therapy time, G's parents continued to give him what he wanted just to make him happy and avoid negative behaviors. Over the months, G reportedly became more and more detached and withdrawn, just using people as a means to get the things he wanted independently.

G's parents justified the screen time by giving him learning games to play. They reported that G was learning a lot from the games and becoming very good at completing puzzles quickly. She wanted to teach him things herself, but G had no interest in reading books or playing with any toys or even interacting with people. His parents had no training in other ways how to work with him, so they were consoled with the idea that G was learning something from the games and videos.

Fortunately, G's parents, like most parents of late-talking children, know their children better than the therapists and doctors. G's mom didn't believe what the doctors were saying, and she also was exhausted from all of these ineffective therapies and from fighting with everyone, including her child. She saw my Waves of Communication videos and started to think about the process from G's perspective, realizing how tortured he was by the therapies. She decided to do something different and try language facilitation strategies instead.

G's mom started by reducing ABA to 24 hours a week and scheduling more fun time with G. She took him to his favorite places, ate his favorite foods, and did his favorite things. She eliminated pressure for him to do anything and just enjoyed their time together so they could feel happy instead of stressed out at therapy. G reportedly seemed much happier to be spending time with her, especially because they were going to all of his favorite places. She noticed that, without her even trying, G started to say more words. That's when G's mom reported she realized that he can talk and that he IS wired for spoken language.

G's parents joined my Waves of Communication program to receive custom coaching from me. I worked with them to intuitively analyze and take responsibility for all their current communication patterns, enabling and prompting habits and even the environmental communication blockages they had unknowingly encouraged. They worked together as parents to honestly examine the activities of their daily lives and identify patterns that are working and those that needed to change.

Then I provided the replacement strategies to make the process of spoken language facilitation easy, happy, safe, and fun for all of them. They gave up facilitating use of the tablet system, flash cards, and prompting immediately and only concentrated on helping G learn to use natural spoken language.

G's parents continued to use the fun experiences they had already scheduled in their day, as well as those activities they did every day as targeted opportunities to facilitate language naturally. They adapted how they talked using what I call "Language Facilitation Talk". This way of talking helps children understand and process every sound of every word that is said. G's parents focused on their new mindset habits, used words that G is interested in, talked using their language facilitation talk strategy and had FUN.

G happily started trying to say new words within days. Within weeks, spontaneous spoken phrases for needs-based and descriptive communication emerged. That's not the only improvement they noticed. Here is what G's mom said after only 3 weeks of language facilitation:

"He is becoming so much more social now and plays with kids all the time, and he hardly has any tantrum and easy to deal with most of any places -- This is how much we have achieved in less than a month since I joined the program, so far so good. — feeling happy."

G's family PROVED that kids talk fast when parents eliminate communication blockages and facilitate language naturally. However, G's initial speech was only emerging with his parents. He continued to shut down his speech whenever therapists pressured him to talk. G's parents told the therapists that he was talking more at home, however, their therapists did not believe their stories, and doubled down on their assessment that G would never speak, and he would need a more complex tablet system.

That's when G's parents decided to quit ABA completely and start the new year in public school. He had started a special education plan (IEP) with detailed services for speech therapy and 1:1 aide due to his behaviors, so G's parents took their plan to the public school in their district. They then set up a meeting with the speech therapist to recreate the plan and focus on spoken language. They specifically requested to stop using the tablet, remove the picture communication goals, and replace them with spoken expressive and receptive language goals.

G's parents faced more external blockages in the process. Initially, the teacher and speech therapist were reluctant to remove the picture system from the education plan, because of G's age. G's parents were quoted that same research that indicates children are typically not able to talk after 6 years old. Fortunately, G's mom was able to share her analysis videos with the whole school team at her meeting. She was able to show them how she used language facilitation and fun to help G learn to use spoken language functionally at home and in the community. They did change his plan and focused on accommodating his need to move and helping him use functional speech in both the classroom and therapy. As a result, G was able to participate in all of his classroom learning experiences more easily and learned to complete his structured school activities independently. G met all his annual IEP goals in 3 months! This year, his is beginning 2nd grade using conversational, sentence-length speech.

In private therapy, G's mom pushed into the sessions and demonstrated for the therapist how, when she eliminated pressure, G wanted to try to fix his speech articulation, and how he refused to work with flash cards but he would talk like crazy in the car. G's mom convinced the therapist to eliminate her high-pressure tactics and work with his feelings and energy instead of shutting him down. Soon, the speech therapist was able to see improvement in his expressive vocabulary and speech clarity. He also began to initiate social interaction with people outside of his family. After 6 months, G's parents stopped private speech therapy completely, and used the money to take mini vacations and swim in hotel pools on weekends.

After 1 year of language facilitation, G is sharing his feelings and eagerly exploring new environments. He is making new friends and learning new things at school every day. His family is spending their time traveling and happily talking about everything and G's language is expanding in ways that his parents never imagined would be possible last year. Every time he reaches a plateau, his parents do a self-analysis, identify the blockages, eliminate them, and progress resumes.

G has come so far, however, there are more steps to go on his language development journey before he catches up with his peers. G's his parents know that he will get there because he makes consistent progress that is noticeable to everybody, every time they make changes and stick with their new habits. G's Mom now has HOPE and CONFIDENCE because she knows that she will have me and the other parents in our lifetime community to help her every step of the way.

The most wonderful thing is that G's progress and his family's success is not unique. It's happening for all parents who become language facilitators.

Waves of Communication Results the First 20 Months

From January 2018 – August 2019, more than 100 families have enrolled in my online Waves of Communication Programs. Here are some results from my first 60 cases of face-to-face, online language facilitation coaching:

The children are all between 2 and 13 years old, and their parents report they have been diagnosed with a wide variety of diagnoses including autism, apraxia, brain malformation, genetic syndromes, global developmental delay and injury from toxins. Some children did not have any diagnosis. All children reportedly passed a hearing screening.

The families are diverse. Many have only one child, and there are also several families with 2 late-talking children. We have a few sets of multiples. Families live in 12 different countries. Most families in the program are bilingual. Many families use English as their second language. The coaching is all completed in English.

Before enrollment in the program, each family attested that they meet the following criteria:
1. The child has been evaluated by an audiologist to be able to hear speech sounds.
2. The child regularly initiates communication with parents - verbal or nonverbal
3. The child can follow basic directions with gesture cues
4. The child has spontaneously made speech sounds at some point in their life
5. The parents are willing to make changes to eliminate communication blockages and facilitate language naturally

Every family received the same amount of time to access to training, guidance, and support to accomplish the following:

- Eliminate prompting the child to say words at home
- Provide language models that the child would possibly use independently
- Facilitate natural spoken language in the moment throughout everyday situations.
- Eliminate child's exposure to ABA or reward-based therapy
- Eliminate all alternative/augmentative communication systems (PROMPT, PECS, Sign language, and picture-based tablet communication systems)
- Use targeted language facilitation talk for 2-3 20-30-minute periods of language facilitation talk per day.

Every child except two (58/60 = 97%) reportedly started to use new spontaneous words consistently within 8 weeks. Parents who participate in my Waves of Communication Lifetime Community group coaching program, report consistent improvement in receptive and expressive language, as well as speech articulation and social interaction.

Interestingly, and not surprisingly, the two families who did not see new language, were also receiving full-time ABA services and/or frequent PROMPT therapy. The children were also both using tablet-based communication systems. In both cases, the parents chose to remain exposing their children to 20+ hours of 1:1 exchange-based learning. The family's videos revealed them clearly using rewards as bribes to prompt their children to use the tablet and to say words. It is of note that in each case, the parents reported that they chose to remain using prompt-based speech training because these methods had been the only ones so far that had elicited sounds or words from their children. They each communicated that they did not trust the language facilitation process.

Many families continue with part-time ABA; however, these families consistently see the slowest progress. Most families who give up ABA see new functional language appear quickly. These families are reporting consistent, functional language growth and successful participation in social experiences such as pre-schools, play-based therapies, and/or activity-based interventions such as sports teams, dance classes, swimming lessons, gymnastics, and music performance.

Many of these children have transitioned from late talkers to chatterboxes. Their parents continue to report amazing wisdom emerging from their little ones as they simply provide functional learning experiences where their children can explore their superpowers and learn with fun. I have been amazed to read the testimonials day after day from parents all over the world who have shifted their mindset to become language facilitators and teach their children to talk faster than I ever could facilitate in 30 years as a speech therapist.

What's really going on is that parents are the best language facilitators. You have the power to teach your child to use natural spoken language that no therapist, teacher, nanny, or anyone else could ever have. If you want to hear your child use spontaneous speech in conversation someday, then you are responsible to teach them. Parents also have the power to enable late talkers to remain stuck in nonverbal communication patterns. If you want to hear your child use spontaneous speech in conversation someday, then you are responsible to eliminate all blockages to their spoken language development.

In the next chapter I provide the structure to help you figure out the root cause of your child's late talking as well as what is going on in your household to block your child's natural communication development. It will be up to you to honestly analyze your household and eliminate blockages. Late-talking children can develop spontaneous spoken language when their parents help release these blockages and then facilitate language naturally. It's that easy.

What's Blocking Your Child's Speech?

This is the chapter where you are going to learn how to get the information you need. You will learn how to analyze your child's history to figure out the root cause of their late talking. You will also learn to look for patterns and habits that cause blockages to your child's natural communication development. I will explain how to complete your self-analysis step-by-step and record your results as you progress through the process. I will also explain how to use video recordings to assist you to be objective and honest in your analysis as well as support your progress.

The Gateways to Natural Spoken Language Development

The following circumstances are necessary for speech to naturally develop. I call them the gateways to spoken language. They are all equally important in the process and blockage to even one of these gateways will result in speech delay in even the healthiest child:

1. Exposure to real people talking to the child at least 2-3 hours per day
2. Ability to listen to and understand people talking
3. Interest in sharing their messages and ideas with other people
4. Confidence in using the mouth for functional language
5. Independence in communicating their ideas using words
6. Freedom to explore their curiosity and interests

When the child has physical ability to talk and remains late-talking, parents need to identify what is blocking the natural language learning process from taking place. These gateways to verbal speech are the key to help parents figure out where the blockage is happening. You can identify all the blockages to your child's verbal speech when you analyze each of these gateways and identify any potentially blocking situations, habits, or circumstances that directly affect your child.

Gateway #1 ~ The child must have exposure listening to humans talking 2-3 hours per day.

Blockages to this gateway occur when the child doesn't have the opportunity to listen to their parents. Late-talkers can be deprived of human talking when they spend most of their waking time alone, with or without technology. Too much screen time limits time to have exposure to humans talking and looking at their face.

Gateway #2 ~ The child must have the ability to listen to and understand people talking.

This blockage happens very typically with children who suffered from middle ear fluid. These late-talking children do not actively listen to adults because they are out of the habit of listening. The temporary hearing loss that happened during the time their ears were full of fluid caused them to be unable to hear and understand clearly spoken speech, so they stop listening. Parents usually give a lot of visual cues when kids can't hear, so these late talkers often shift their focus away from listening, which is difficult, to visual learning during these times. Instead of listening to the words their parents are saying, the child learns to watch the parent and respond to their demonstrations. Then they start to imitate and use the same visual cues and demonstrations that their parents used to help them understand. If the hearing loss happens for a few weeks or more, children easily fall into the habit of watching their parents instead of listening. If they have success with their new visual language, they will start to use other nonverbal behaviors on their own. This is how they shift into nonverbal language.

Parents can perpetuate this blockage by talking fast. Late-talkers who are not good listeners can't learn to speak clearly when parents are talking fast. Remember, these children are just starting to be able to hear spoken language after a period of hearing loss. Even if they have been exposed to speech, they didn't hear it clearly enough to learn all the sounds in the words. All late-talking kids find it difficult to listen and focus on speech when it is too fast. This makes them give up on trying to learn spoken language quickly because it is too frustrating.

Gateway #3 ~ The child must have an interest in sharing their ideas and messages with other people.

Blockages occur in this gateway when the late talker avoids listening and "tunes out" the people who are talking to them. This can happen for many reasons. Take a moment and think about what causes you to stop listening to someone who talks to you a lot.

Emotional trauma, any kind of anxiety, fear or PTSD that happens in a child's life can cause them to be afraid of interacting with others. Equally as blocking, a lack of confidence in speaking skills and shyness causes many children to avoid interacting with others. This is the exact situation faced by every late-talking child, especially as they get to be older than 3-4 years. If they are not successful, many children avoid socially communicating with other people which blocks their ability to learn from them.

Many late talkers lose interest in listening to people talking because they are only hearing a lot of the same repetitive words, prompts, questions, and/or vocabulary they have heard 1000 times. Nobody likes to pay attention to the same teaching over and over, especially if we already know the subject matter.

Many late-talking children have been "trained" in structured therapies and by parents that their favorite actions like spinning, humming, running, lining things up, or moving in their seats are not desired. This causes the late talker to isolate themselves to escape and experience the things they love away from those who judge them or correct them all the time. Some late-talking children actively avoid engaging with their parents because the primary language that they hear every day is yelling about behaviors or nagging to say words.

Gateway #4 ~ The child must want to try to use their mouth to say words correctly.

This blockage happens even in children who have no physiological problems with their oral motor muscles. Some late talkers appear to have difficulty moving their mouth because they are not able to imitate speech sounds, even when prompted. It is rare for a child with functional eating skills to have difficulty moving their mouth only for speech. Children who have good fine and gross motor skills often choose to favor physical communication and use their hands and body as their communication tools instead of their sounds. A late-talking child who prefers to use behaviors and demonstrations to communicate will resist saying sounds and words that have no functional purpose for them because it is like "work". Other children are "perfectionists" and refuse to try to talk because they don't think they can say the words perfectly.

Shy, or anxious late-talking kids develop feelings of inadequacy and anxiety from having to repeat saying sounds and words over and over to get a reward. This inadequacy blocks the late-talking child's confidence to try to talk on their own. This results in the child resisting any pressure to try to say words because they see it as a test that they could fail or just repeated work.

Children with severe blocks in this gateway are commonly given a picture or tablet-based system because the child consistently refuses to imitate words and the therapist cannot make progress in verbal speech without this skill.

<u>Gateway #5 ~ The child must want to try to communicate their messages using words.</u>

This gateway becomes blocked when children are in the habit of depending on others to communicate for them. Many late talkers who had some physical illness fall into the mindset that other people are responsible to say words for them because they have needed assistance for other things like walking or eating. Parents fall into the mindset of enabling children to be extra needy, even after they have learned to do skills. This blockage is perpetuated when parents are stuck in the habit of anticipating the child's needs and guessing what they want by their actions. Other parents block their child's speech by over-scheduling the child's life. Late talkers who have blockages to this gateway frequently perform actions and wait for their parents to respond with talking.

Complete blockage to this gateway is caused when children become dependent on other people to prompt them to say words. The prompt-dependent child one who only talks when prompted and uses behavior to communicate their independent messages. The prompt-dependent late-talker is not a verbal communicator, even though they say words. These kids learn that the only time to talk is when other people tell them what to say. For all of their own independent communication, they continue to use behavior.

The first thing every parent should know is that prompting children to say words, even repeatedly, will never teach them to use natural language. Prompted speech is simply a behavior, such as a sign, point, or facial expression. Children respond to prompting only to get the reward for saying the word or to be compliant with your request to talk. This is not the same as independently using words to communicate ideas.

Children who are prompt-dependent will develop the ability to use words to communicate needs, however, they will consistently choose to use their nonverbal system communicate their feelings and unique ideas.

Gateway #6 ~ The child must have the freedom to explore their curiosities and interests.

Children learn how to use the words they know naturally as they find ways to communicate the ideas that they imagine in their minds. All children learn about the things they love by watching and listening to everything in their environment. Children require assistance from their parents and teachers to nurture their curiosities and create safe opportunities to explore them. This is how all kids develop an interest in learning more about a topic. When late-talking children are interested in a subject, they will automatically want to learn the language to talk about it and try harder to say the right words.

Blockages to this gateway occur when the late-talking child is not 100% invested in the language facilitation method, the teacher, or the environment where they are supposed to be learning to use spoken language. Parents can easily identify blockages in this area when you analyze your child's reaction to the intervention.

Blockages to a child's curious exploration are indicated by the following behaviors:

- Your child does not like to go to the session and shows anxiety when you approach the building, even after you have been there many times.
- Your child does not look at the therapist's face without prompting.
- The therapist must reward your child to sit with them or complete their tasks.
- Your child is not using any spontaneous vocalization in the therapy session.
- Your child is eager to leave the session and find you.
- YOU don't like how the therapist is talking to or behaving with your child, even if your child is ignoring the therapist.

If a child doesn't like doing the intervention, or even being in the same room with the interventionist, then whatever they are doing is obviously not going to help the child overcome something that's challenging for them. If your child doesn't feel the therapy is easy, happy, safe, and FUN, they will be too distracted trying to feel better to learn anything.

Blockages to a child's curiosity and imagination can only happen from outside triggers. Late-talking children who receive a lot of pressure to follow directions and prompts often naturally retreat into their "own world" whenever they have a chance. They do this so they can think about and imagine whatever wild and wonderful things they want without someone stopping them.

Sensory regulation issues affect a child's ability to explore new things, even when they enjoy them. Many late-talking children have difficulty processing different kinds of sensory input and this causes an ongoing feeling of anxiety. To avoid feeling anxious, late-talkers try hard to avoid the things that trigger uncomfortable feelings. Sometimes, late-talking kids avoid the whole experience of listening to people talking to them because doesn't feel good. The speech they hear may sound irritating to them in some way. Some late-talkers report getting headaches when certain people talk to them or sing. Children with sensory regulation issues often learn from trial and error, that behaviors such as moving, listening to sounds, and looking at things in a certain way can help them regain control over their anxiety and feel better.

Many times, the self-regulating input that children seek involves activity looks like "off task" behavior, such as wiggling, spinning, flapping hands, and looking at things in a line. Therapists often report to families that their child's behaviors are "distracting" the child from doing the learning task. The opposite is true. When therapists stop children from self-regulating their feelings, they cannot learn new things because they are too distracted by their anxiety. Often, the child is not even aware they are doing the movements and they learn much better when allowed to self-regulate. It is other people who are distracted by the child's behavior.

Get Yourself Organized

The first thing you will want to do is get yourself organized. I recommend that you create in a digital space where you can, store all your notes, your analysis videos, as well as documents from professionals that you work with. I recommend you create a digital folder in the Internet cloud using one of the many free platforms available. These online services typically provide enough secure cloud space for parents to keep all your videos as well as an ongoing document to record your notes, questions, and progress. They also have easy options for sharing your documents and videos via email, which can be super-helpful when you are coordinating your child's team and even sharing their progress with Grandma. Use your favorite search engine and investigate the different options for yourself.

The first document you should create is your language facilitation journal. This will be an ongoing document that you keep adding to as you progress through the process of helping your child move from where you are now to spoken language success. If you are serious about your efforts and responsible with your notetaking, this document will serve you well.

These notes will save you time and mental energy. Instead of writing multiple emails to everyone on your team from scratch, you will be able to cut and paste your notes for easy communication. Journaling is a wonderful way to keep your mindset in check too. If you ever get triggered by seeing some chatterbox showing off at a birthday party, you can go back to your notes and celebrate how hard you and your child have worked to overcome obstacles and you will remember how much better you feel today than you did before you found out that you CAN teach your child to talk. Your journal is your own place to record your journey as a language facilitator parent as much as it is to record your child's challenges and successes. In fact, by the time you spend a year taking notes about your language facilitation journey, you will probably have gathered enough notes to write your own book! By the way, if you do write a book about your journey, I will be the first to buy it.

The Analysis Process

Now that you understand what is necessary for natural spoken language development, you need to figure out why your child is late talking. You're going to have to use the information you have now to identify any physical root causes, as well as all situations or circumstances, that are blocking your child's gateways to natural spoken language development.

Here are the gateways again:

1. Exposure to real people talking to the child at least 2-3 hours per day
2. Ability to listen to and understand people talking
3. Interest in sharing their messages and ideas with other people
4. Confidence in using the mouth for functional language
5. Independence in communicating their ideas using words
6. Freedom to explore their curiosity and interests

Identifying Physical Root Causes

The best possible overall wellness is necessary for natural language learning. Any child who is feeling unwell will always focus their energy on physical and/or emotional healing before they can effectively learn to spoken language. Parents must identify and resolve any root physical blockages to the gateways to spoken language and maintain the child's best overall wellness for language facilitation to be effective.

The process begins with reviewing your child's health history. Starting when you were pregnant, write down all the possible situations, interventions, illnesses, or occurrences that may have affected your child's physical development in any way. Make a chronological list of any "stand out" events and list your child's approximate age. It is not necessary to take the time to dig through your records, just think about it together with your partner and write a list of any physical things that could have affected your child's development in any way.

What you really need to think about, instead of diagnosis, is the physical challenges your child has experienced in life, not just the stuff that the doctor told you. List the challenges that you KNOW your child's body and body and mind have been focused on healing. If your child is/was late walking, they likely focused on walking first, because they must move freely to explore for natural language to develop. If your whole family was focused on healing from a big illness or developing eating or walking skills, many gateways are blocked due to the common focus being on basic survival. There is no extra energy to focus on language facilitation or learning. The unwell child may be isolated in bed.

Additionally, an unwell child may be too exhausted from healing to pay attention, listen or share their thoughts. A late-walking child is typically interested in trying to learn the act of locomotion and getting to things on their own. Until they have freedom of movement, they can't explore well enough to know what they are missing to learn about. They also become passive and wait for others to do things for them. Both situations block a child's ability to experience new things and develop their curiosity which is necessary for natural language development.

Review each item on your list and consider which of the gateways to spoken language were/are blocked. Then, write down the current status of that blockage. Have you found a resolution to this problem? Then mark it FINISHED, or if you like color, mark it GREEN. If you are in the middle of treatment that is seeing consistent progress mark the blockage as RESOLVING, or color it YELLOW. If you are unable to understand how to resolve the blockage, mark it ONGOING and color it RED.

Identifying Environmental Root Causes

Your child's everyday environment needs to have a lot of practice opportunities for natural speech to develop. This is how the gateways to verbal speech are kept open and clear. What could be blocking your child's exposure to looking at, hearing and understanding people talking? If they are not able to talk with others for at least 2-3 hours per day, what are they listening to instead?

Starting again at the time of your pregnancy, make a list of any significant events or ongoing situations that have caused any significant change in your family. Even if these things seem to affect only the parents, write them down, because parents are the primary language facilitators, and when they experience issues, these issues affect the child. Big changes in family income can affect kids because it affects the whole family emotionally. Significant events such as moving to a new house, family members coming and going from the home, childcare switches, encounters with animals, and even big trips can cause a child to stop spoken language development. Any kind of trauma can really affect these gateways. A very common symptom of PTSD in children is selective mutism.

A late-talking child's fears can severely block spoken language gateways. Parents need to identify and understand their child's fears to help them overcome. Write down all the kinds of things that your child avoids and think about why your child avoids them from their perspective. You must figure out what it is that causes their fear. This fear comes from worry of shock, surprise, uncertainty or being threatened. Think about what surprises your child does not like. What makes them feel threatened? A late-talking child's need to feel safe from the things they fear will always block spoken language. Think about how your child's unresolved fears are blocking verbal speech gateways.

Review your list and analyze how any of the significant changes in your family may have affected your child's spoken language gateways. Consciously decide the current status of each blockage you identify and label it, using the color system.

Before You Move On

Physical and environmental root causes should all be either resolved (green) or Ongoing (yellow). If your list has one or more issues highlighted in red, I advise visiting a holistic medical practitioner or licensed mental-health practitioner for comprehensive evaluation so you can investigate specific intervention methods to resolve these issues.

Identifying the Child's Self-Blocking Habits

Starting from birth, list any behavior patterns, including verbal and nonverbal communication behaviors, that you have noticed throughout your child's development. Make a chronological list and identify any behaviors that your child uses a lot. Write down helpful communication behaviors as well as those you are concerned about. Write down any behaviors you have seen more than 10 times even if you don't understand why your child did/does them.

Your late-talking child may prefer to use behaviors to communicate instead of verbal speech. Late-talkers use problem-solving and trial and error to find the behaviors that parents understand consistently. Some children try to spell words, point to the pictures on their videos, or bring objects to their parents to try to communicate their messages. For example, a child may bring their cup to parents to request a drink. Other late talkers get in the habit of being independent instead of relying on others to help them get the things they want. When this happens, children are consciously avoiding talking. This blocks their progress. Think about specific times when your child appears to be avoiding using words to communicate their messages.

Other late talkers develop behaviors specifically to block you from teaching them. Look at all your child's regular communication behaviors that they do on their own and see how your child may be blocking their own spoken language development gateways. What does your child do frequently when you try to work with them or teach them something? Think about times your child blocks you from talking to them and write them in your notes.

Many late talkers try to control the communication system of the household. They become very focused on their little "missions" and become in the habit of making sure everyone does things "their way". These late-talking kiddos can appear to be very resistant to listening to other people. This happens because they don't understand verbal speech well and they don't want to be wrong or make a mistake. They may just ignore you or tell you to stop talking because they don't want to listen. Controlling late talkers become in the habit of directing everyone around them to do things or say things. This is how they know you understand their messages. Think about ways your child is trying to control your household and how these habits are blocking natural speech gateways.

Identifying Blockages Within Your Household

Many late talkers get stuck in these nonverbal communication habits due to other people's repeated influence. Consciously analyze any habits or long-term situations created out of necessity, because these habits can cause blocks to form slowly over time. Chronic or long-term illnesses cause families to develop habits that previously made life easier, however, now are no longer needed. Parents must do a lot more to help children when they are very young, and these requirements continue longer when children are unwell and developmentally delayed. As late talkers get older, parents often get stuck in the habit of trying to guess and anticipate their child's needs. They continue to do things for their children long after they are capable to do these things for themselves. This blockage enables the child to give up their responsibility to learn to talk. The child becomes dependent on the parent to interpret their ideas and communicate their messages to other people. Consciously think about ways that you enable your child to rely on you to communicate for them instead of empowering them to take responsibility for communicating their messages. Think about specific situations that you find yourself talking for your child instead of helping them learn words for the situation.

As I noted before, many late talkers develop their own way to communicate using gestures and noises and behaviors. Parents often habitually respond to the behaviors without facilitating any spoken language. Sometimes parents respond to a child's nonverbal requests simply by complying without talking. This blocks a huge opportunity to facilitate language. Some late talkers use undesired communication behaviors such as screaming, tantrums, or physical aggression. Parents often respond to these big behaviors with yelling or punishment instead of facilitating the words for the child's feelings or intended communication message. Think about the specific times you have encouraged your child's nonverbal communication habits and write them down.

Identifying Blockages from Outside Influences

Boring, repetitive, annoying, and stressful intervention methods, cause children to remain stuck in nonverbal communication. These intervention methods may start to work well at the beginning as long as it is easy and fun and there are big enough rewards. However, most kids outgrow reward-based systems quickly. The smart late talkers eventually figure out that the repetitive activities are not making their life better, so they try to get out of them. Then they are taught that they need to "do the job" or face restriction of their fun. The reward turns into a bribe and the teaching transfers into everyday struggle to get through so many tasks in a day. They are expected to learn to do things as they are directed, in the same way each time, and follow all the rules just like a factory worker. This completely blocks the child's natural interest to explore their surroundings and engage in talking opportunities with a variety of people. Think about the times you have asked your child to do something to get a reward and consider how the spoken language gateways are blocked by this habit.

It often happens that late talkers already have learned or memorized whatever's been presented to them and they're just bored. They've done it already a lot of times, they know it, and they just don't want to do it again. Sometimes late-talkers are demeaned, put down, or bullied by people around them. Unfortunately, this can happen too from teachers, administrators, and even therapists. In schools, clinics, and therapy sessions everywhere, late-talking children are being asked to do things they do not find enjoyable and they are expected to do these things frequently and obediently. Many children are placed in classrooms where there is chaos every day. Think about the times in your child's life when they are forced to do things that they do not want to do.

Consider what they are expected to do that is not easy, happy, safe, or fun. Consider how these outside influences block your child's gateways to spoken language.

Using Video for Analysis

Video analysis is the method I recommend for parents to objectively see and hear the truth about your family's current communication situation. Watching your recorded situations later will allow you the time to separate yourself from the emotions of the moment. This way you can have a clear mind and view the recording multiple times. This is the presence of mind necessary for you to objectively analyze the interaction from all perspectives. This is analysis is how you can discover what is blocking your child's speech and language.

Video analysis is the most important tool parents can use to help you see progress along your language facilitation journey. Video analysis is the key to identifying all communication blockages instantly. If you have completed your analysis notes, then, you already have ideas about what is what might be blocking your child's speech. If you have read this far and still have no idea what could be blocking your child's speech, then honest objective video analysis will reveal them to you. When you understand and eliminate all the blockages to your child's spoken language development, you can see progress immediately. If you don't find ALL of the blockages, your progress will be slower.

<u>Use your smartphone to record short videos of communication situations in your household.</u>

- Your child alone doing what they love the most
- Your child showing you how to use a toy they know how to work very well
- Your child requesting food and drink from you, and also from others

- Your child requesting help from you and from others in your family
- A time you do not understand what your child is trying to communicate
- A selfie video (your child looking at themselves) while you talk about something that they love to talk about
- You with your child while you talk with them about something fun you did together
- You and your child reading a book together and playing with toys together
- Your morning dressing routine and typical mealtime
- Moments when your child seems to be frustrated and have meltdowns
- Your child interacting and communicating with other children

Video Recording Tips

Nobody has to see these videos except you. Let the camera capture everything. You need to be able to see behaviors and hear the words with the best quality possible.

Sometimes children interact differently when they know they are being recorded. So, it is wise to both record situations when the child is interacting with the phone and also gather recordings from an "outside" perspective. This way you can see the difference. You will also be able to analyze how your child interacts with you, the camera, as well as with other people. You can also ask someone else to record your child and invite them to interact with the person holding the camera. Alternatively ask someone else to silently record your interactions.

When creating all recordings, the focus should be on capturing the entire communication situation so you can analyze it later. Set the record button and forget the camera. If you don't have someone else around, you can prop the phone in the corner of the room or and let the video run while you play and talk together. If your child is having a meltdown at home and you want to record the situation (as long as your child is safe) go ahead and take a second to silently hit the record button on your phone and set it nearby. Then attend to your child.

You will be glad to have at least the audio recording and your child will wait for you if you don't call attention to your recording process. If your child is frequently frustrated and upset, you'll want to have this recording. It can be very enlightening to watch how you respond to your child when they're having a meltdown.

When you are setting up recordings, be sure there is enough light in the room and there is limited background noise. Try to turn off the volume on your child's show and talk about the characters instead of talking over the video. Make sure the microphone of your phone is not obstructed as well. It can be frustrating to have captured a great moment and end up with poor quality recording. It doesn't take much effort to get clear pictures with most smartphones.

Try to keep recordings between 30 seconds and 4 minutes long. This is often enough typical communication, interaction, time to make an analysis. Shorter videos are easier to share via the Internet with family members and professionals who work with your child.

Using All Resources Available to Find the Answers You are Looking For

This is the time for you to be 100% honest with yourself. You will see things in these videos that will make you happy and things that will make you cringe. All of it is true, and it is your job as a language facilitator parent to take responsibility for it all. Now that you understand that you have all the power to teach your child to talk, you can't ever honestly rationalize, justify, or project any reason for your child's speech delay onto someone else. Besides, if you are blaming your child's late talking on someone or something outside of yourself, then you are giving away your own power to fix the problem.

Read through your notes so far and make a mental note of the highlights. By now, you should have at least a suspicion of one or two blockages happening in your household at this moment. Think about how you are feeling about yourself and your child right now. Consider your mindset as well as your child's attitude about talking. Make a few notes in your journal about what you think you may see when you do your video analysis. Your notes will provide you with the clues to look for when you review your videos.

Watch each video one by one and go through each of the following sections to identify clues. In your notes, give the video a title to describe the action and the subjects such as "Reading books Mom and Joey" or "Reading books Joey alone". Under each title, make notes for each of the following sections:

Section #1 List all of the communications you observe.

Identify and write down all the different behaviors, sounds, or words that your child used independently and follow it with your interpretation of the meaning of that communication behavior. For example, you observe your child handing you a book about sharks. Your interpretation of this communication behavior is "my child wants me to read this specific book about sharks." Remember, every behavior is communication, so even a small gesture like this is a communication attempt that you can use to facilitate language.

Watch your child solve problems and learn how to do things on their own. Notice the things that your child has learned how to functionally communicate very well. If they are not using words to communicate, what are they doing instead? How do you "know" what they want? Watch their behavior on the videos and notice how they use facial expressions and/or physical movement to communicate. Figure out WHY they are doing the actions they are using to communicate and use your intuition to identify what they mean by their actions.

Your video analysis will provide you with good practice for spotting and interpreting all your child's communication during everyday life. Notice the communication behaviors your child does repeatedly. These are the components of their "language". Pay close attention to identify any behaviors your child does to intentionally avoid listening to you or make you stop talking. Look for any behaviors that are clear avoidances to try to say words. These are obviously blockages.

Section #2 – Analyze your own communication habits.

Review your notes from previous sections and look for potential patterns and habits that you suspect might be blocking your child's gateways to spoken language development. As you look through the videos, you will notice that you are doing and saying some things repeatedly. These are the patterns and habits of your family communication structure. They are your current "method" to get your child to talk.

As you view yourself on the video, analyze your language facilitation strategies. Look for your execution of all the tricks, and tips that you have incorporated either consciously or subconsciously into your everyday life and notice how effective they are. Notice the patterns of your language models. Write down the words and phrases that you hear yourself saying frequently.

Think about how your speech affects your child. Look at the situation from their perspective. Are you helping them evoke their superpowers and empower them learn new words, or are you noticing any patterns that could be blocking the gateways to spoken language development? You will likely find both in your videos. Especially notice how your activity potentially enables your child to avoid talking and rely on you to say words for them. That's a very common blockage.

Section #3 – How is everybody feeling?

Look at your child's facial expressions, body language, and actions and write down how they appear to be feeling on the video. Consider the context of the situation the situation from your child's perspective to understand what causes them to feel the way they do. Watch the whole situation to understand what is happening consistently to make you and/or your child avoid talking or listening to you. Look for signs of sadness, disinterest, anger, or annoyance. These feelings are easy to see on video. Look for the patterns of behavior that cause the feelings you observe.

Pay attention to how you feel when you watch these videos. If there is anything you observe that makes you feel worried or fearful, it's wise to view the situation objectively as a problem-solving exercise. Consciously think about what you could do to immediately change your own habits and think about how you can make a shift in some small way. Remind yourself that the next time you watch videos, you will feel better, because, now you understand what you need to change. If you can make a commitment on the spot to do some small thing better from now on, you will be on your way to becoming a powerful language facilitator fast.

Section #4 - Watch out for the times that your child wants to talk.

Observe the things that your child focuses their attention on. Identify patterns of behaviors that they do to feel happy and the things that make them feel upset. Notice the vocal patterns your child is producing when they feel emotional and listen very carefully to see if they could be tries at saying words. Notice the things that trigger your child to make a vocalization. Observe if their vocalization is a try to say what they just heard, or if it is something they are trying to say on their own.

While you are watching, say the words out loud that you suspect your child would say. Say phrases to communicate their feelings such as, "oh no, my ice cream is all gone!" or "I love you mommy". Hear yourself say the words out loud so you know how your child will hear them when you model them next time you have a similar experience. It will be good practice for your face-to-face language facilitation time.

Section #5 – Make notes about how your child is learning.

Parents can learn a lot about how your child learns by watching them do the things they love. You can observe all your child's developmental skills this way. In fact, it is the method that professionals use to evaluate children for delays. Notice the tasks that your child finds easy and those that they struggle with. Notice what makes them frustrated and how they solve their problems.

Observe your child through their problem-solving process. Identify what happens when your child succeeds at something that they try hard at and what happens when they fail. Analyze their surroundings to see what causes them to push through barriers and what causes them to give up. Watch your child's behavior carefully to discover what it is about their favorite activity that empowers them to push through tough times and try hard to learn new skills. Parents who discover their late-talker's favorite things, can ignite natural "superpowers" to try and do things they otherwise would never attempt.

Situations that Cause Blockages Due to Habit and Mindset

The following are some of the most common habits that block spoken language development
- Prompting speech with rhymes and fill-in-the-blank
- Singing the same rhymes and songs over and over without modification
- Talking to the child when they are not listening
- Using screen time, speech therapy, or outside sources to teach the child without being 100% involved in the process
- Ignoring a child's feelings and forcing or bribing them to do things they don't like

- Anticipating needs and then asking the child to say words
- All day "Quiz Show" of questions and never ending "testing" to identify and say words
- Worry and focus on problems and/or the future instead of targeted strategies
- Facilitating use of an alternative, nonverbal, exchange-based communication system such as sign language, tablet picture systems, or picture exchange.

Write down any of these situations that are happening regularly in your child's life.

If you have truly spent time with conscious thought and use honest analysis of the information you have written, you should now have a clear picture of what caused your child's late-talking and what is blocking the gateways to spoken language development.

ACTION ITEM

Parents who want to see the fastest improvement take dedicated action. To help you get started, I offer you a challenge called Swapping the Prompting. Parents are encouraged to eliminate prompting and other blockages from your household completely for 7 days and replace the ineffective strategies with language facilitation. There is a video on my YouTube Channel to take you through every step of the challenge so you can see new focus and engagement in 7 days or less.

Hundreds of parents all over the world have taken this challenge already and many have heard new words emerge spontaneously even the first day! Here is one of many emails that I have received from parents who have swapped their prompting for language facilitation:

Dear Marci,

I just wanted to reach out to you and let you know that I've taken on your Swapping the Prompting Challenge and have seen results immediately with our 7-year-old son.

He seems to be listening to me more and we are having more back and forth interactions between us. The interactions feel natural and relaxed. He is using more varied vocabulary, picking up on words and phrases I'm saying, and he's started using them without prompting.

It's only been 1 day. Wow.

As you know, this is not easy, it's the biggest challenge of my life, and I often feel discouraged and stressed and worried about it all. So, watching your Waves Of Communication videos gives me some much needed motivation and hope that we can facilitate his language learning.

I just wanted to give you some feedback and say a big THANK YOU.
~ V.C.

The Swapping the Prompting Challenge is a very powerful tool and I encourage EVERY family to take advantage of this challenge. Please follow this link to find the step-by-step process video on YouTube: https://youtu.be/g37Pk06bRLQ

Language facilitation strategies will only work for parents who consciously eliminate blockages and continue to analyze their progress. Parents who find themselves stuck at any time in your language facilitation journey, should return to analysis and identify any blockages that have reappeared.

Language facilitation is a process with a lot of ups and downs. Parents must be vigilant in ongoing analysis to continually keep the gateways for spoken language development wide open. Simply put, you will not see progress if you neglect your responsibility for eliminating blockages to your child's spoken language development. However, when you swap your prompting for language facilitation, your child can learn to use spontaneous, spoken language faster than speech therapy. Parents are proving it all over the world.

Reach and Teach Your Child the Words They Need

This is the phase of your language facilitation journey where you will learn how to "reach and teach" your late-talking child how to use the words they have memorized. This process opens the gateways to spoken language learning and sets up the perfect little opportunities throughout your day to naturally teach your child the words they need. Reach and teach is also how you will help your child shift from avoidance to desire when it comes to spoken language learning.

In this chapter, I will discuss the strategies to join your child in situations where they feel most comfortable and secure without pushing them away. You will learn how to connect with their energy and feelings and encourage them to respond naturally and want to learn from you. I will show you how to make sure your child willingly focuses on every word that you say so they understand you clearly. This mindset shift is necessary to help your child learn speech from you.

Reach and Teach is the process to help your late-talking child feel safe allowing you into their own private mental space and then to gently encourage them to share their ideas with you. When late-talking children feel safe to try to talk and share their ideas without judgement, their confidence builds, and they try harder. This is what is necessary for a late-talking child to shift their mindset from being a nonverbal communicator into a self-empowered, proficient talker.

Step #1 - Analyze Language Learning from Your Child's Perspective

Parents must develop the habit of looking at the life from your child's perspective to understand their current mindset. You need to use all your senses to understand every communication your child makes with both verbal and nonverbal communication energy. This exercise will help you relate to your child and understand their language learning experience.

It will help you "get in their head" and encourage them playfully, to share their wisdom using verbal speech. Complete the following analysis activity to help you understand your late-talker's mindset.

<u>Observe your child while they are doing their favorite, self-directed activity.</u>

It doesn't matter what your child is doing but it must be self-directed. Consciously observe every action they do for 5-10 minutes without calling attention to yourself. Notice how your child is using all their senses to explore the activity. Make a note of their reactions to the stimulus they are experiencing in the immediate environment.

Listen to what your child is hearing. Notice how they react to what they hear the sounds, words, and/or music. Analyze what auditory stimulus causes them to pay more attention and what causes them to recoil or go away. Look at the things that your child is visually focused on. Observe the way they are using their eyes to examine things and try yourself to see the object from the same visual perspective. Watch your child's reaction when they look at and examine things, situations, and even people.

Objectively observe your child when they don't see you watching them. This way you can notice what kind of external visual stimulus is spontaneously catching your child's eye without you doing any intervention. Notice the type of stimulus that is causing them to react in the same ways. Pay attention to what visual stimulus is keeping your child's attention as well as the things that distract them away. Notice the kinds of things your child avoids looking at.

The same kind of analysis should be completed for all the 5 physical senses. Consciously analyze how your child uses touch, smell, and taste to enjoy, learn about, and share their favorite experiences.

Experience the things your child loves in exactly the same way they do.

A great way to see things from your late-talker's perspective is to try them for yourself. If your child enjoys laying on the floor and watching the ceiling fan, try it yourself with an open mind. Try it first when your child is not in the room. Quietly relax and observe all the details of how it looks. Notice the movement and the light. Feel the breeze from the fan and the temperature of the room. Listen for any sounds the fan is making. Say out loud exactly what you are experiencing using complete sentences.

If your child always asks for macaroni and cheese with ketchup on it, smell that food, take a bite, and notice how it feels in your mouth. Objectively analyze exactly what it tastes like and say it out loud using descriptive words like sweet, sour, salty, etc. The words you are saying out loud are the words that your child needs to learn if they want to share the experience using spoken language.

Experience the same things when your child is not around. Do not "push in" or modify their experience in any way. The object is for you to take some time to think about and learn how they experience the things they love. You may have very different preferences about the things your child enjoys, and it is key for you to avoid trying to change your child's opinion, or even impressing your preferences upon them. If you suspect your child's favorite drink of two kinds of juice mixed together will taste awful, you won't be tempted to share your opinion if you taste it on your own.

Look for patterns in the experiences your child enjoys independently.

Once you have observed your child during their most enjoyable experiences and you have experienced the things that they enjoy for yourself, then you need to take the next step and tap into your intuition to figure about your child's WHY. The objective of this whole exercise is to figure out what are the different kinds of stimuli that cause your child to feel in different ways. Late-talkers use their behaviors to communicate their basic needs, ultimate desires, and deepest feelings. You can understand why your child does the things they do when you analyze and understand how your child feels during the actual experience. You will also uncover your child's superpowers.

When you view your late-talking child's nonverbal communication from their perspective it is easy to spot their nonverbal communication "tricks". These patterns and processes are the late talker's "language". Consider your child's everyday experiences to obtaining and eating food. When your child is hungry, what series of behavior experiences do they create to ultimately get food in their belly? How do you know your child is even hungry? When you consider your child's basic communication experiences from their perspective you can think about the words that your child would, could, and will say, after you facilitate the language. These are the words your child is highly motivated to learn how to use functionally, so they will learn these words fast.

Use your intuition to understand your child's messages.

When people experience things together, natural intuitive communication happens naturally. When we look at, listen to, smell, taste and feel things at the same time as another person, we share that experience. In these moments, the right words always come out naturally. ALWAYS. When you share experiences at this level with your child, you will always know what words to say because you are experiencing the same thing. You simply use the words to describe what you are feeling in the moment and your child hears the words while they are feeling the same way.

A parent's intuitive communication connection with their child is the most important "sense" for language facilitation because it is the best way to see life from your child's perspective. This way you can easily model for them the words they want, need and FEEL right in the moment. When your child is focused on their favorite activities and enjoying them with you, then you can teach them the words they want to communicate those feelings. Here's an easy example: When your child has a happy face right after they taste some ice cream, you say "Yummy! Ice cream tastes yummy!" This is how your child relates the word yummy with how they feel in the moment of tasting the ice cream.

The natural intuitive connection is strong between children and their parents, especially their mothers. There is research going on right now at Yale University involving fMRI imaging of mothers and children. The project, led by Dr. Joy Hirsch, has collected images of observed both mother and child's brains lighting up in the same areas when mother spoke the child. So, in the 3D world it is measurable. This intuitive connection is how you as parents know what your child is wanting almost before they do. You are already "in tune" with them. This is also why in many cases it is only the parents who can understand the late-talker's nonverbal needs-based communication and respond to all their feelings, happy and sad. It's also how parents understand nonverbal children's humor.

<u>Avoid expecting your child to say the words you intuitively "know" that they know.</u>

Parent blockages sneak in when parents expect the child say out loud messages that they intuitively perceive- but they haven't taught the child how to say verbally. The child's blockages happen when they start to expect parents to continually guess their needs and communicate for them. This is the mindset of a late-talking child that can keep them stuck in nonverbal communication indefinitely. Late-talkers have been communicating intuitively with their mothers since before they were born. Children who are highly controlling and/or anxious are often resistant to talking because they are literally afraid of people talking to them. They intentionally avoid talking and will sometimes try to use their intuitive connection in addition to behaviors to try to get others to say words for them. Parents who fall into the habit of always guessing what their child wants without facilitating the language for it often find themselves trained by their child to be their interpreter.

<u>Children can only make big changes and try new things when they feel their best.</u>

Parents need to incorporate the sensory experiences your child loves into every activity you do so that every activity feels easy, happy, safe, and fun. Language facilitator parents reach children with the activities that make them feel happy and they teach them the words they need in the moment, throughout the entire experience. So, if your child loves to move their hands or smell everything before they eat it, you need to honor those preferences to help your child feel comfortable as you guide them to change their communication.

Some late-talkers life experiences have left them so blocked that they don't enjoy sharing their favorite time with other people. They may use their unique activities to escape from parents and anyone else who is restricting their happiness. In all cases, parents must never try to adjust, adapt, or push-in to their child's independent fun uninvited. If your child is not interested in sharing their experiences with you, start by observing them and making comments about the things they react to.

Step #2 - Facilitate joint attention

Your first attempts to share experiences with your child should be parallel instead of cooperative. Don't try to interfere with your late-talking child's independent actions, unless they are unsafe. Just let your child know that you just want to be in their space and share their energy because you want to watch and see what they do. Tell them you are just looking. Keep your hands to yourself and Don't touch their materials. Quietly watch them as they do what they love and don't say anything until your child initiates some communication with you. They may just look at you and keep playing or they may try to push you away. If this is the case, tell your child you respect their space and tell them that you will be watching from across the room. You child must be comfortable with you being nearby. Watch when they smile, watch when they get frustrated. Watch whatever they're doing, and really understand what they're experiencing while they're doing this thing that they love.

<u>Be your child's cheerleader and biggest supporter.</u>

If they are independently trying to solve a problem, watch and encourage them through the process from a distance and praise every small accomplishment. Tell them you love the cool and unique things they are doing and remind them how smart they are to figure out the things they do. Use a gentle voice and limited words just loudly enough so you are sure that your child hears you, but not loudly enough to disturb your child's fun. Children typically love when their parents say nice things about what they do independently, so you will likely observe your child stop and look at you with a smile. This means your child is listening. Make a note of how you approached your child and what it was that seemed to trigger their new engagement with you. Every child responds differently, however parents can easily learn how to engage with their kids when they eliminate pressure.

To avoid intimidating or prompting the child, the language facilitator parent uses simple language to describe only their own actions as well as the child's. Comment on and celebrate the child's behaviors and respond with simple language that the child can understand. "You kicked the ball in the water! That was a big kick. OH NO the ball is stuck. I can't get it! Let's go and get a net. We need a net to get the ball back. I can scoop it out. I want to play kicking ball again. We need to be careful, right?"

<u>Empathize with your child's feelings and honor their emotional needs.</u>

Whatever communication the child initiates, verbal or nonverbal, you should respond by acknowledging that you understand their communication by responding to all their requests. If the child is requesting something you are not willing or able to give them, you must tell the child that you are unable to comply and immediately communicate your empathy for their disappointment. "I know you want to have another cookie, but we are on a 2-cookie rule in our house. BUMMER! No more cookies! How about a hug and we go kick the ball instead?"

Some late-talking children may need repeated attempts before they will consistently trust parents enough to come out of "their world" and share their favorite experiences. Even after a successful and fun interaction, the late-talking Child may retreat into their own space again to process their feelings. Always allow your child the space the need to process their feelings. Parents may need repeated attempts with different activities and even less pressure.

Step #3 – Turn your child's attention into curiosity.

Once your child starts responding to your words by looking at you and smiling at you, this means you have your child's attention. The next step is to try to increase the time they allow you to engage with them.

Follow your child's lead to get them to notice you.

Imitate exactly what your child is doing in a parallel play situation. Use your own toy, food, or object and try to experience the same thing your child is enjoying by imitating them. Let your child observe you slowly try to do the same actions they have done while you talk through your own process. Your child will observe you imitating them instead of asking them to do something. This is how parents can regain your child's trust that you won't try to take away their toy, change their play or stop them from doing their favorite things just the way they want. Additionally, your child will see you modeling the words for your actions that are identical to what they did themselves. This is how the language facilitator parent "reaches" the late talker so they can make the connection between the actions they recognize and the words they know.

Here is an example of how that looks: Let's imagine the late-talking child has a plastic ball and he is sitting in the corner throwing the ball repeatedly into the corner. The ball bounces on the floor and then he catches it. Every time the ball hits the tile floor, it makes a certain "squeak" noise. The child has thrown the ball for 10 minutes without stopping. The parent may think it is annoying, however, Mom notices that every time the ball squeaks the child giggles.

Mom walks over near the child and when the ball hits the floor, the mom says "squeak!". The child looks at the mom and hesitates because he thinks she will make him stop. Mom says, "do it again" and points to the wall. The child throws the ball again and mom again says "squeak!" then the child giggles and looks at mom. Mom says "you throw ball - squeak - and then she giggles saying I like it! Do it again! Mom continues to watch and say the one word that makes him giggle until the child is interested in looking at the mom. Then he looks at her and throws the ball, as his way to ask her to "say it again".

Then, Mom says "I throw ball", gets a different ball, and throws it against the same wall. Her ball makes a different noise. Mom says, "pop" when her ball hits the floor and then she giggles. Mom looks at child and says, "my ball pop" Then she gestures for the child again to throw his own ball and she says "squeak". "Your ball squeak" Then she throws her ball and says "pop - my ball pop". The child giggles with both. They continue to throw their balls side by side and Mom says the noises. Then, after a minute. Mom stops and waits for the child to initiate the next action.

<u>Attention to faces is important for spoken language learning.</u>

Making sure your child focuses on your face as much as possible while you are talking. They don't need to stare at your face, or even look at you the whole time, however, it is important that they periodically look up from their toys to acknowledge that they are listening to you. It is YOUR responsibility to attract and keep your child's attention and encourage them to look at your mouth. Hold objects near your mouth when you talk about them. Look in mirrors so your child is not intimidated by face-to-face pressure. Do not prompt your child to look at you.

Instead, encourage them to look at other people's faces by pointing out the facial expressions and feelings of people in your household as well as the people you see in pictures or watch on video.

Another way to attract and sustain your child's focus on your face want to look at you more while you are talking, is to talk about the things your child is doing, holding and looking at, in the moment. Use your senses to model phrases about those things your child is experiencing right now and watch for them to look at you when they "agree". This is how you get visual confirmation that your child is paying attention. Eye-contact may only be brief acknowledgement that the child is still listening as you tell your story. This is enough. Many children

The best way to get a child to look at you is to say out loud the words for their feelings, their emotions, their opinions, their attitudes. Watch their reactions to different stimuli and say the slang phrases that kids in your world use to share their experience. Say word such as Uh-oh. Bummer! Yuck. Love that. That's cool. Wow. No Way! Children really enjoy hearing adults say these words and they want to use them to be like other kids. Late-talkers enjoy learning these words and often, the fun phrases are the first ones to pop out spontaneously. These phrases also help children sound more natural and engage with other people socially.

Spoken language is about so much more than just labeling stuff and requesting. It's about sharing our feelings and opinions. Late-talkers often show their feelings with actions such as flapping hands when they are excited or covering ears when they are afraid. In these moments, model words to express their feelings so they know you acknowledge them. Show empathy to your child when they have a meltdown and tell them the words to communicate their frustration.

Regain your child's attention with silence.

If you are talking to your child or reading a story and you suspect your child is not listening, here is a super cool trick. Just stop talking. If they stop what they are doing and look at you when you stop talking, then they were listening. But if your child doesn't notice the change, it means they weren't listening to you carefully enough to pay attention. In these moments, you must use one of those strategies to get their attention again with visual confirmation that they are engaged with you. Many parents of late-talking kids send me videos of them telling stories, giving directions and asking questions when their children are not even listening to them. You must attract and keep your child's attention throughout your whole language facilitation situation that you choose your activity because otherwise, you're just wasting your breath.

Step #4 - Help your late-talker love to learn speech and language from you.

Facilitating joint attention for language learning is important, however, it is just the start. Parents of late-talking children have a responsibility to help their children change from disliking talking to thinking speech is a good idea and wanting to try hard to improve every day. As all parents know, just because a child is listening, doesn't mean they will respond to your language facilitation efforts. Sometimes, children choose not to respond or "shut down". This situation only happens for two reasons.

Always make tasks easy for your child.

The first reason that causes late talkers to shut down is that the child feels like the task is too challenging and they don't have support. Even when parents know that a child can do a task, it is the child's lack of confidence that causes them to shut down. They will consciously avoid, cry, whine or give up on the communication opportunity if they think it is too hard. So, you must assist your child with every task, whether it's a talking task or a non-talking task. Whenever they hesitate you must acknowledge their need for assistance and offer to help them do it. Stepping in and doing the task for the child enables them to avoid trying in the future. To build their confidence, help them work through the problem and celebrate their successful outcome. Most late-talkers are very confident in the things they know how to do. They often do not try to do things if they feel they will make a mistake. When you help them succeed with your assistance, they will have more confidence to try next time.

Show your child how useful speech can be.

Another reason that a child refuses to engage is that they do not see any personal benefit from the situation. Whatever reward is offered, is not worth their required effort. If a late-talking child is not interested, they often use their lack of speech to silently frustrate their communication partner. Most late-talkers are great at waiting for their desires to be anticipated or guessed by others. If they don't want to do something, then they just don't. Some late talkers learn to be obedient, even when they aren't having fun. They learn how to do only the minimum amount of "work" to satisfy the request and keep you happy. Children love to make their parents happy because when parents feel happy, it reflects in the whole family's experiences.

If it isn't **FUN**, it **ISN'T** fun.

It's wise for parents to always acknowledge your child's wishes to stop any activity, because if they're communicating that they are done, then they're done. If they are having a negative experience, and showing it via behavior, you must acknowledge their feelings and help them process the situation before trying to return. You can't just tell them to stop the behavior.

This is important. any attempt to try to redirect a late-talking child and force them to comply without acknowledging their communication a blatant disregard for their feelings and independent ideas. This situation is a common blockage for spoken language development. When children's feelings are disregarded, it causes them to withdraw more and be more independent. Parents can help children adapt to challenging situations by preparing them beforehand with education and experiences to educate the child about what they can expect. During activities, limit expectations for pressure situations that can cause anxiety.

If a child is finished listening to you, it is likely because they are overwhelmed by their emotions. Look at the situation from your child's perspective to understand why they are feeling negative. Help them process these feelings by talking about them and offering a solution that will help your child regulate and focus again. Unless you take these steps, the child will continue to try to escape.

Teach your child the words to empower themselves.

If your child does walk away from you or refuse to do anything that you ask them to do, you should be facilitating language for that activity too. You can use phrases such as: You don't want this. It's too hard for you right now. You are done. Not right now. And my favorite, No thank you. Whenever you see a sour expression, your child rolls their eyes, crosses their arms, or stomps their foot, this is their way of communicating their feelings. Language facilitator parents model the right words their child would need to communicate their disappointment. If you want your child to seek you out and communicate their feelings to you no matter what, then you need to teach them the words they need to do so instead of ignoring their messages.

Step #5 - Modeling language using Language Facilitation Talk.

Children can only learn how to use the words they know from hearing examples of how those words are used functionally. Before a parent can realistically expect a child to use spontaneous spoken language, they must have provided many, many hours of language facilitation models without any expectations for talking. The real language teaching starts when the late-talking child begins to listen and focus on parents' words, and they respond with their own verbal and nonverbal communication methods. This is how parents know the right words to teach them. With language facilitation, the idea is to provide your child with the right words, the right way, at the right time so they learn what to say the next time they are in the same situation.

What is language facilitation talk?

"Language Facilitation Talk" is the secret to unlocking a late-talkers speech. This method of talking presents the late talker with speech and language models that are representative of the words that your child will say when they become a talker. Once you have reached your child, and they are able to listen to you when you are having fun, language facilitation talk is the best way to provide the speech models your child needs to learn to use spoken language functionally. You're going to learn why this kind of talking works and how it helps kids learn natural language. You're going to learn the structure of language facilitation talk and you're going to learn how to incorporate it into your life starting today.

Why is language facilitation talk so effective?

Late talking children missed exposure to clear speech and language while their blockages were in place. To compensate, the late talker has been focused on visual and physical communication. Therefore, they don't know how speech works. Late-talkers learn primarily by watching and are not in the habit of listening. All the talking they have heard has not been effectively processed because the child didn't listen to every word being said. They pick out the words they have memorized and use visual cues to fully understand the message.

Language facilitation talk helps parents demonstrate how to use the words kids need to use and want to say because the words that are facilitated always apply to the current situation. Words are always modeled in phrases, so children can see how to construct functional phrases to demonstrate how their memorized words can be used for all language purposes, instead of just making requests. The speech is super slow and clearly spoken, so even children who didn't hear or pay attention to speech before, now can understand every sound in every word. With language facilitation talk, it is easier for children to follow and contribute to a whole conversation instead of single phrases and requests.

When other people intuitively interpret the late-talker's feelings and then use words to describe them, they learn that using speech is more efficient than the non-verbal communication behaviors they have been using. When parents model easy to understand speech about the fun things your child loves, late talkers listen because they want to hear you talk about the things they love. Children also want to learn the words they need for everyday activities such as getting dressed and interacting with their favorite people. Your child will pay attention and learn how common words are used when they hear them spoken clearly during their everyday experiences. Parents need late-talkers to pay attention to them, so they can model the language that their late-talker missed.

Late-talkers still have not learned their first spoken language. Their first language is the nonverbal system they have developed. Language facilitation is like teaching a second spoken language. Many of the ideas behind this language learning method resemble philosophy of immersion foreign language learning. The difference is, your late talker is learning their first spoken language.

The structure of language facilitation talk

Parents should speak slowly and clearly enough for your child to hear every single sound in every word. The rate of speech should be as slow as you can speak while still stringing sounds together. Think super-slow or 5 times as slow as you usually speak. Do not take breaks between sounds in a word. Smoothly say each sound in the word and stretch out sounds that continue such as /s/ and /f/. Use inflection and animation in your voice to grab attention.

Kids often pay attention to the inflection and animation voices they hear on tv and videos. Using enthusiastic, inflection is important so your child pays attention, however, don't take the voices over the top because the goal is to facilitate functional language that you child can use with everyone.

All words should be spoken in phrases to help the child understand how the word is used in context. No single words should be repeated unless you are playing with words or singing a song like "shake, shake, shake your sillies out". If your child is using fewer than 20 words consistently, you should speak 2-3-word phrases. 3-5-word phrases are a good length for kids who already have needs-based speech. Phrases must be short because late talkers can't hear every sound in every word in long phrases. They are likely missing a lot of sounds in fast talking.

Even though the late talkers can frequently demonstrate understanding when parents give them directions, they are not listening to every sound in every word. Slow talking allows the late talker a chance to hear speech before it passes them by.

Use the same words repeatedly, however, change the phrase to allow the late talker to hear the word used in different contexts. For example, when a child requests a cookie by saying "cookie", model phrases such as: "you want cookie, cookie please, yummy cookie, my cookie, chocolate cookie, cookie all gone.

Slowly spoken phrases should have 1-second breaks between them to allow the late-taker the chance to hear the words, apply them to their situation, and respond. the breaks between phrases is important to continually assess if your child is listening to you. When parents continually talk, they are not able to know if the child is understanding everything. Give the child a chance to respond to every statement you make.

Incorporating language facilitation talking in your life

Language facilitation talk is most effective in 20-30 minute "sessions". Ideally, a family should try for 8-10 hours per week of super-slow language facilitation. I encourage every family to start with one session per facilitator, per day. As each language facilitator becomes comfortable and confident with your language facilitation talk, they should add sessions, one-by-one, up to 3 sessions per day. Every language facilitator should commit to completing at least one 30-minute language facilitation talk session every day. Even in a really busy day, parents must make a commitment to provide super-slow, super-careful talking.

A helpful strategy is for each parent to choose a very consistent activity that you spend 20-30 minutes helping your child do every day. Think about your entire daily routine and identify the personal care activities, household chores, and community trips that you experience almost every day. Dressing, bath time, bedtime, and car ride time are very common choices. If you have a daily commute, this is perfect Language facilitation time.

Use your language facilitation talk when you are out in public during times your child is struggling with communication. When they shut down, tantrum, or otherwise appear frustrated, slip into your language facilitation talk. You can use it right in the moment to help your child focus on every word you are saying as you talk them down from their meltdown. Whenever you see your child struggle, immediately analyze the situation from your child's perspective, acknowledge their feelings, and use your language facilitation talk to recover from any meltdown anywhere. It's an amazing tool.

Other perfect times to use language facilitation talk are the fun activities that are initiated by your child. Watch them and use the reach and teach strategy to do exactly what they're doing. If they're tearing paper, lining up trains, or they're twirling in the swing, you do the same thing so that you can experience it for yourself. Then provide short phrases for the actions you are taking and make comments on the child's actions.

Use short phrases to describe every step and every aspect of what you are experiencing. Allow your child to watch you and listen to you talk about your experience so they can relate to what they are doing. With your language facilitation talk, your child hears you say all of the specific words that relate to their choice of experiences in context, used functionally. It's the best way to learn how spoken language works. You say the exact things, you are doing, e.g. I turn the Knob, I jump high, flip the switch, it's so big, Mom eat chicken, I bite my apple, it tastes yummy, you have yellow shirt, I have blue. Say the words that tell the story of what you are doing, including your reaction to the experience.

Another great opportunity to practice language facilitation talk is to encourage your child to teach you something. Ask them to show you how to do their favorite activities and explain what they are doing to show you using super slow phrases. Make sure you tell your child when you don't understand them and repeat everything they say clearly so they know you understand them. When children are motivated to teach you something, they will try harder to say words to explain themselves.

If the child struggles with finding the words they need, have them show you, and then you give them the words for that explanation.

To explain playing trains, you may ask your late talker to show you how to make the train go. Phrases sound like put the train on the track, connect the train, push the train, it goes up the hill, watch the corner, uh oh, train crashed. Slowly tell the story that you watched them demonstrate and ask them if you can have a turn to "try it". Let them nonverbally guide you how to do it if they want to and use words for their guidance such as: put it here, push it, give me that, it goes this way. They're going to use their nonverbal way to show you and demonstrate it then you use your language for that too.

You can use your language facilitation talk to model phrases we need to learn. Try saying phrases such as: "You are pushing the buggy. Can I push it? Mommy is pushing buggy. Is this how you push it? Thank you for teaching me. Now I understand. I can do it all by myself!" Remember to leave spaces between your phrases. This will give your child a chance to process and respond to every phrase that you say and keep their focus on your talking while you tell the story of the experience.

Creating the Optimum Language Facilitation Opportunity

Easy. Happy. Safe. and FUN. These are the components of the most successful language facilitation opportunities. First, the task must be easy for the child to do with your assistance. Your child should be able to complete the activity with 100% success if you are there to support them. So even if it's a mildly challenging task that your child does not enjoy, you can make it easier for your child by providing more assistance. It is not wise to combine language learning with other physically challenging tasks like potty training. For language facilitation to work, your child must be focused on listening to your speech instead of solving a problem.

The opportunity must be happy. Overcoming a challenge or accomplishing a task creates feelings of success. Many late-talking kids love to hear praise. So, help them learn how to solve little problems and complete little jobs followed by heaps of praise and celebration. Use phrases such as "we did it" "You are amazing" and "I am so thankful for your help!" Children love feeling so successful that they can help others. It is empowering for late talkers to share accomplishments. When you talk about these experiences, it will surely make your late-talker happy.

You want your child to use you as a resource, to come to you for help and know that you are a to help them learn all the things they want to know how to do, including talking. The language facilitation opportunity must feel safe. When children feel fear or anxiety from pressure to perform, these feelings block their ability to listen to and focus on your talking. When the blockages to the gateways of verbal speech are eliminated, children feel safe to try to talk.

Natural spoken language learning can also happen from problem-solving negative situations in the moment. For example, children can learn the word hurt very quickly when a parent facilitates it in the moment that they get a skinned knee. That is definitely not a fun situation, however the interest in learning words to communicate their big feelings will he high in these moments. Children desperately desire to communicate when they hurt or when someone hurt them. Facilitating language in negative situation is always a huge benefit to a child's overall health and safety.

The most important component of every language facilitation opportunity is that it must be FUN for both the child and the language facilitator. This means that the language facilitator must take responsibility to find ways to have fun in every situation, or at least look at it from a positive perspective. Most late-talking kids are resistance to talking, and the situation must be super fun to facilitate engagement, interest, joint attention, and ultimately the motivation to try to talk.

If it isn't FUN, it ISN'T fun.

Of all the tips in this whole book, that's all you really need to remember. I recommend writing it on a sticky note and posting somewhere you will see it frequently. When you intuitively connect with your child, you can tell if they are having fun or not. When you are in the moment, you will feel it in yourself and you'll see it in your child.

It is important for the language facilitator to have fun in the process, because, just as you intuitively perceive your child's feelings, they feel yours too. Parents' lack of trust in themselves, and in their abilities creates a block in the fun. Even if you don't outwardly share your feelings with anybody, your actions will reflect your overall energy and your child can feel that more strongly than anyone else. Every strategy that you make up for every opportunity that you take should be fun for you as much as it is for your child. Because, if it isn't FUN, it ISN'T fun. You have to release your expectations, worry and fear so that you can all have fun with this process.

Using Your Child's Superpowers to Facilitate Language

Every child has superpowers. Language facilitator parents learn that the best way to get late-talking kids excited about speech and add rocket fuel to their language facilitation journey is to talk about their superpowers. A child's superpower is the skill, talent, or activity that they find easy, happy, safe, and fun EVERY time they do it. They receive a lot of personal satisfaction from doing their favorite activity. When children enjoy an activity, almost to the point of obsession, they practice that skill frequently and become very proficient. Most late-talkers focus their energy into activities that highlight their amazing skills, such as visual arts, construction, movement, and problem-solving and nonverbally negotiating ways to avoid talking!

Alternatively, when children lack confidence in any skill, they are typically not interested in working hard to try to succeed, especially if the task seems challenging. Late-talking kids can spend a lot of time in their minds. They think in pictures more than language and make up movies in their head. They also develop superpower memories because people ask them and show them how to do things over and over while they are being directed through life. When late talkers are alone, they spend a lot of time thinking and processing the input they have received throughout their day and replaying the images to experience the feelings again.

Most late-talkers are aware that they do not know how to communicate the messages the visual messages and feelings they think about. Language facilitator parents help late talkers feel confident talking about the things they are thinking about in the moment, so they try to actually say the words out loud and share their wisdom.

The ability to tune out anything and avoid even the loudest noises is a real superpower. Late-talking kids who have difficulty regulating their sensory systems, become very good at tuning out the world and independently finding things to help themselves feel better. They are better at self-calming when they have free access to input that makes them feel better.

Often late talkers develop super skills from repeatedly doing the activities that generate the feelings that they want to experience. Late-talkers who are regulated can enjoy social interaction and this is necessary for spoken language development. Language facilitator parents always provide children with access to the sensory input that makes them feel comfortable while they teach the child words to describe the actions and feelings as their child is experiencing them. When parents speak out loud and relate to the feelings their children are thinking about, it helps them learn how to communicate their feelings verbally instead of with behaviors.

Most late-talkers have access to videos, and they learn quickly how to find topics that interest them. When they are alone, watching these videos repeatedly, late-talkers have the capacity to memorize volumes of visual and auditory information. Without spoken language, the only way to extend the fun they experience is in their own mental time. Some late talkers with access to technology become very skilled at using it.

They learn how to find videos in different languages for example. Language facilitator parents talk about the things that the child has been watching and relate the information to real life experiences. They teach their late talkers to use technology to create their own videos and make the voices themselves. This helps late talkers share the information they enjoy with others using technology and their own speech.

Most late-talkers don't like change. In fact, they can be very, very good at controlling the environment because they're so good at problem solving how to avoid what they don't like. They develop the superpower of teaching others to understand their nonverbal language and manipulating others to do what they want, including to stop teaching them and go away.

Late-talkers learn to communicate when they want to be left alone by creating behaviors that are off-putting. Some late talkers become really controlling and good at ordering people around without using any words at all. These are the children who I call the future CEOs. Language facilitator parents empower controlling children to use words to order people around.

Some children develop amazing physical abilities. In the process of enjoying their freedom of movement, they learn how to do gymnastics, dance, and sports like running and swimming with excellence. Other kids develop superpowers from their love of taking things apart and building things. Superpowers such as drawing, playing musical instruments, and creating physical art like sculptures with clay or dough are common, as well as cooking.

Through their repetitive activities, late-talkers develop the neurological pathways for becoming super-skilled at their favorite activities. It really has to do with focused attention, motor movement and repetitive practice. Language facilitator parents encourage their children to participate in these activities and facilitate the language that goes along with the whole environment.

All kids want to say the words that surround their superpower. They're good at it. It's always easy. They're successful every time. It's always happy. They have no fear of their superpower. It's always safe for them. Even if they do something you think is dangerous, they think it's safe. They will take risks and try new things if they feel this way. That's why using superpowers always triggers natural speech.

Superpowers offer perfect language facilitation opportunities because they are always easy, happy, safe and fun. You just encourage your child to explore them, reach them when they allow you into their world and facilitate the words they need. That's how easy it works.

Super-smart language facilitators think about other situations in their every-day life that require similar skills and abilities to their child's superpowers. Then, they teach their children to do functional, useful tasks using the same skills. For example, late-talkers who like to move a lot, may be good at shaking up a milkshake. If your child likes to run, teach them to run to the mailbox safely and fetch the mail. If your child likes to problem solve and push buttons, show them how to help you prepare food and do laundry. Test their strength by giving them things to carry and stamina through completing the whole task. Give them fun challenges during these activities and you will help them develop life skills that they will keep forever.

At the same time, language facilitators can connect and relate the same "shake it" vocabulary that you facilitated while your child was shaking a jar of vitamins to hear the rattle, as you do while they mix the milkshake.

Use your language facilitation talk appropriately in both situations and your child will shift from ignoring you to begging you to talking more. It happens during their superpower time and during the activities you want and need them to do with you every day. When your child learns that they can feel easy, happy, safe and fun playing and talking together during your everyday activities as they do when they have spent time on their own, your late-talker will definitely choose to spend more time listening to you talk. That's because they LOVE you more than anything. You are their parents!

Online Resources to Support Your Language Facilitation Journey

There are more than 200 videos on my Waves of Communication YouTube Channel.

Parents who are interested in specific strategies, examples and demonstration of language facilitation talk can find video resources on my YouTube channel. There are many examples of language facilitation opportunities that you can adapt and use today. New videos are uploaded weekly, so be sure to subscribe and hit the bell notification so you are aware of any new content.

If you have seen progress with your child's speech, I'd love to hear your feedback. You are welcome to join me every Thursday at 2:00 PM Eastern time, for my live Q&A session on my Waves of Communication page. Every week, I answer questions from parents who are trying language facilitation and provide strategies to respond to the many different situations that arise in families.

Please consider posting a review of this book and share your experience with language facilitation on my Waves of Communication page or Amazon.

Language facilitation and the information in this book is directly in contrast with what many speech therapists, doctors, and ABA professionals are telling parents every day. If you have found that the system has led you down the wrong path and you are finally seeing success with language facilitation, your experience may empower another parent to go with their intuition instead of what professionals are telling her like you did.

You may help another Mom find hope, like the other parents in my Waves of Community do for each other every day. If you are interested in reading about other parent experiences, and sharing your story, please visit Waves of Communication on Facebook.

Thank you so much for reading my book! I hope you have a ton of FUN with your child as you start to hear their natural speech emerge. I'm sending you all the love in my heart because you got this! You CAN teach your child to talk faster than speech therapy.

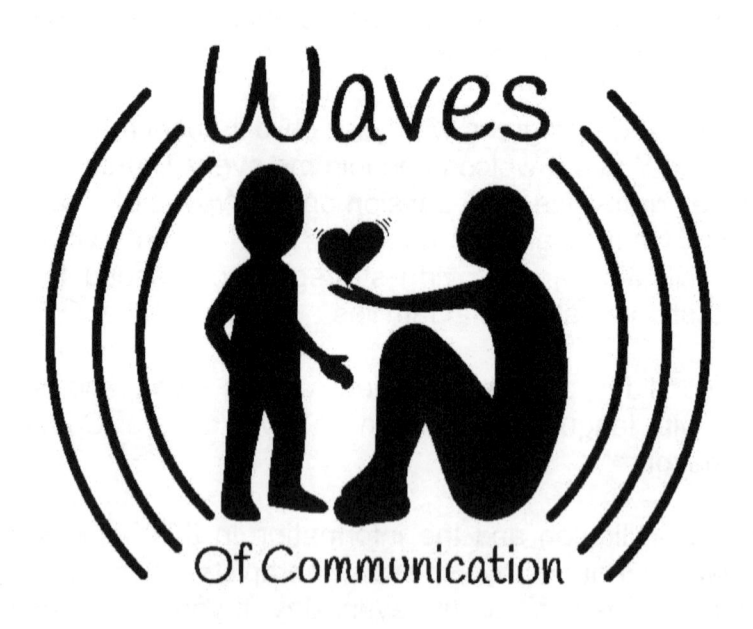

About the Author

Marci Melzer earned her M.Ed. in Speech-Language Pathology from the University of Virginia in 1990. She has always been interested in providing "out of the box" intervention methods with clients who demonstrate challenging communication behaviors.

In the late 1990's Marci presented multiple presentations and workshops at national conferences across the United States speaking about innovative and evidenced based interventions designed to maximize outcomes with children who have been diagnosed with autism spectrum disorders.

After only 10 years as a speech pathologist, Marci developed and grew a large practice with 30 therapists providing early intervention services in the Chicago area. However, due to Illinois state early intervention system failing to pay her for more than $250,000 for services already provided by her employees, Marci had to file bankruptcy, close her company and go back to work as a staff speech therapist.

As a newly single mom raising two young children, Marci earned her living and honed her skills worked as a contractor speech therapist, filling positions in public and private schools, hospitals, residential facilities, outpatient clinics in Illinois, Arizona, Nevada, and Florida. While maintaining a private practice with clients in their homes. Marci's most recent contract work has been with the Florida CMS system to provide speech therapy for children the Early Steps Program.

In 2015, Marci began studying energy healing, diet, and mindset practices, and has cured her own physical health issues via lifestyle changes and plant-based medicines. Her doctor has officially cleared her from requiring pharmaceutical medication which she was told by multiple doctors that she would have to take for the rest of her life.

Through the healing process, Marci developed and practiced her intuitive abilities. She has, through her experience and intuition, developed a keen ability to analyze a family's communication situation and identify the reasons children are choosing not to try to develop and use spoken language as their primary communication method.

In practice with her clients, this intuitive ability has helped Marci break down the target expectations for language development into realistic, easily achievable, FUN goals that parents can integrate easily. The strategies are effective because they are designed to take advantage of the parents natural teaching ability and follow what the child wants, creating ease in communication energy movement.

Marci's mindset work is foundational for the success of her clients. She strives with every connection to help parents overcome their own mindset and energy blockages, as well as empower them to make the small and consistent changes they believe will take them toward their dreams of helping their children learn to use words.

Marci meditates daily and connects to universal energy through the tools of astrology, tarot, and oracle cards to get information about the best interventions for her health and mindset work. Occasionally, her clients Marci to use these divination tools to assist them, however, it is for fun and to give us topics to think about in our discussions. Marci relies on her knowledge as a speech-language pathologist to guide her clients as they facilitate spoken language success with their late-talking children.

Marci is now offering, her Waves of Communication Parent Coaching Programs to parents all over the world. Parents from 12 countries are taking advantage of this unique the opportunity to learn from her knowledge, experience, and intuitive insight. Marci is helping parents transform themselves into Language Facilitators and their children are talking.

Are You Ready to See FAST Progress?

Does the idea of helping your late talking yourself resonate with you? Do you believe you have the power to help your late-talking child learn to use words to communicate their wants and feelings? Are you prepared use loving guidance and to hold positive space for your child to develop language on their timeline?

Language facilitation is positive, systematic, and proven to be effective. If you are interested in receiving hand-holding guidance throughout your entire language facilitation journey, you might want to consider working with Marci as a client so you can receive custom training.

Within our lifetime Waves of Communication Community, parents are educating and supporting each other, and they all receive the empowerment they need to see the kind of language they have dreamed about. If you are ready to learn how to make a shift in your teaching, I have an online class designed to help you get started. This class will show you how you can transform from a being parent who is worried for the future and relies on others to "fix your child", into an empowered Language Facilitator parent who confidently teaches your child to use the words they need to secure their future yourself during your everyday life. Visit WavesofCommunication.com to learn how you can start your child's communication transformation today.